Pandemic Solidarity

'Just what we need so desperately in this moment. How we come out of this pandemic will shape the future of humanity. Now, as never before, we have to break the deadly logic of capital. A beautiful and important book.'

John Holloway, author of *Change the World Without Taking Power*

'In the midst of a global crisis, we must listen, learn, and build with people from around the world – the essays and insights collected here help us do just that. A crisis is a turning point, and this valuable book can serve as a guide to a better future.'

Astra Taylor, director of *What Is Democracy?*

'Our better angels live just around the block, everywhere. These stories teach us of the enormous potential for love and resistance in a world threatened by apocalyptic capitalism.'

Mike Davis, author of *City of Quartz*

'Mutual aid, solidarity and commoning become most visible during periods of deep crisis. This is when the structures of the state and of capitalist markets not only fail to address the emergency situation, but they often show their complicity in making it worse. When solidarity is revealed to the majority as the practice that makes a difference, it is as if society en masse were to whisper in our ear its desire to evolve: "I want to evolve, I want to evolve, but my evolution depends on you," says society. And again: "Make this relational care embedded in solidarity the new gravitational point around which a new world is built." This book listens to this whisper and inspires us all along the path to social change.'

Massimo De Angelis, author of *Omnia Sunt Communia: On the Commons and the Transformation to Postcapitalism*

FireWorks

Series editors:

Gargi Bhattacharyya, Professor of Sociology,
University of East London

Anitra Nelson, Associate Professor, Honorary Principal Fellow,
Melbourne Sustainable Society Institute, University of
Melbourne

Wilf Sullivan, Race Equality Office, Trade Union Congress

Also available

Reinventing the Welfare State:
Digital Platforms and Public Policies
Ursula Huws

Exploring Degrowth:
A Critical Guide
Vincent Liegey and Anitra Nelson

Pandemic Solidarity

Mutual Aid During the Covid-19 Crisis

Edited by Marina Sitrin
and
Colectiva Sembrar

Foreword by Rebecca Solnit

First published 2020 by Pluto Press
345 Archway Road, London N6 5AA

www.plutobooks.com

British Library Cataloguing in Publication Data
A catalogue record for this book is available from the British Library

ISBN   978 0 7453 4317 4   Hardback
ISBN   978 0 7453 4316 7   Paperback
ISBN   978 0 7453 4320 4   PDF eBook
ISBN   978 0 7453 4319 8   Kindle eBook
ISBN   978 0 7453 4318 1   EPUB eBook

Typeset by Stanford DTP Services, Northampton, England

Contents

PART I   GREATER MIDDLE EAST
(ROJAVA, TURKEY AND IRAQ)

PART II   SOUTH AND EAST ASIA
(TAIWAN, SOUTH KOREA AND INDIA)

PART VI   SOUTH AMERICA
(ARGENTINA AND BRAZIL)

List of Figures

Series Preface

Addressing urgent questions about how to make a just and sustainable world, the Fireworks series throws a new light on contemporary movements, crises and challenges. Each book is written to extend the popular imagination and unmake dominant framings of key issues.

Launched in 2020, the series offers guides to matters of social equity, justice and environmental sustainability. FireWorks books provide short, accessible and authoritative commentaries that illuminate underground political currents or marginalised voices, and highlight political thought and writing that exists substantially in languages other than English. Their authors seek to ignite key debates for twenty-first-century politics, economics and society.

FireWorks books do not assume specialist knowledge, but offer up-to-date and well-researched overviews for a wide range of politically-aware readers. They provide an opportunity to go deeper into a subject than is possible in current news and online media, but are still short enough to be read in a few hours.

In these fast-changing times, these books provide snappy and thought-provoking interventions on complex political issues. As times get dark, FireWorks offer a flash of light to reveal the broader social landscape and economic structures that form our political moment.

Fireworks

Foreword

Rebecca Solnit

There's a remarkable sentence in Marina Sitrin's introduction to this exceptional collection of portraits of mutual aid around the world: "Decisions were never based on where there was known solidarity groups and networks, as I assumed they are everywhere." We have often heard about mutual aid and grassroots relief projects as things that suddenly spring up, like mushrooms after a rain, or occur in particular circumstances out of the efforts of particular kinds of people. This might be about defining mutual aid and solidarity too narrowly or not looking hard enough; they are indeed everywhere and always have been and they are what sustains us, the anti-capitalism even in what are supposed to be the most capitalist nations and cities. Layla Ali tells us, in this book, "Social solidarity in Iraq existed since long ago before the pandemic. I am used to giving away money for donation each month, even before the pandemic, I also take care of two orphans that I have never met …"

The generosity without strict rules of reciprocity within families (after all, though you may decades later take care of the parent who cared for you, the contract is unwritten and unenforceable), the work many religious groups do, the work of non-profits and networks dealing with everything from human rights to climate change come to clean up the mess of free market capitalism as ideology and actuality. In fact, capitalism is constantly failing – producing desperation, destruction, alienation – and anti-capitalism comes to undo what it has done and does.

Thus, in many places around the world, civil society, sometimes as the kindness of neighbors and other individuals or casual networks, sometimes as already organized groups, did work that was necessary because of the failure of governments to limit the impact of the virus and meet the needs of people in this crisis. And there were many emergent groups as well, overcoming the requirements of physical distance to find practical, moral, and emotional connection. As Turkish writer Seyma Özdemir shares through her interview with the Kadıköy Solidarity Network, "We know each other from various democratic organizations, workers' unions, collectives and various political groups in Kadıköy. We contacted each other, got organized very fast and announced Kadıköy Solidarity Network within four days of the Ministry of Health acknowledging the first positive case."

More than ten years ago, I wrote a book about how people respond in disasters, prompted in part by the terrible fictions that had caused real deaths in 2005 after Hurricane Katrina breached the levees and put four-fifths of the city of New Orleans underwater. Institutional authorities, egged on by journalists failing to tell stories of real crimes by police and white vigilantes and credulously repeating false stories about crimes by the black residents, from the city's mayor to the governor of the state of Louisiana to the federal government, assumed that New Orleanians would behave monstrously in the chaos of the flooded city – would become criminals, and their efforts were focused on containing – imprisoning – the people trapped in the city and treating them, grandmothers, babies, and everyone in between, as the enemy. Even in those circumstances people inside the city took care of themselves with bravery and generosity, and others outside the city eluded the authorities to sneak in and bring supplies and medical care or bring people out in boats.

I was equipped to recognize what was happening – both the ugliness of institutional authority's failure to take care of people and demonization of those people and the beauty of ordinary people's generosity, creativity, solidarity and bravery – because I had been preparing for the hundredth anniversary of the 1906 earthquake in my own city, San Francisco, where similar things had happened. As they had in earthquakes in China, Nicaragua, Argentina, Mexico, Italy and so many other places and in so many other kinds of disaster, including wars and economic collapses, around the world.

What was, in the end, remarkable to me was not that ordinary people took care of others, but two things. One was that they knew how to self-organize and that horizontal democratic means were what worked, over and over, in place after place. The other was the joy they seemed to find, even in the worst of circumstances, in finding the agency to act, and the communion of acting together and finding a connection that can be hard to find and feel and have recognized by others in ordinary times. This too is reflected in this book: "Solidarity makes people feel incredible emotions nowadays," says one of the Turkish sources. "My phone number is one of the contact numbers on posters. We hear this sentence many, many times: 'You reminded us that we are human-beings! I heard this both from those who have resources to share and those who are in need. This is so real! Solidarity makes us human beings indeed."

That joy speaks to who we really are and what we really want, and those are not things that advertising, mainstream media and entertainment, privatized art such as the purely personal novel, conventional cynicism recognize or profit from. Yet another voice in this book: "In the modern/colonial world, we are disciplined to be lonely. The oppressors call this loneliness 'individuality.' They make us believe that the body of an ideal individual is impermeable and intact." We do not want to escape work for leisure: we want to escape meaningless and exploitative work and overwork, but not meaningful work, work that has tangible benefit, that connects us to others, that has meaning. We want the agency that comes from this work. We want to be members not just of romantic relationships or families but of civil society.

This knowledge is itself powerful. If this is who we want to be, if this is who we are capable of being, then ... at the beginning of the millennium Arundhati Roy famously said, "Another world is not only possible, she is on her way. On a quiet day, I can hear her breathing." In disaster she is all around us, and we are her, and so the question is how to stay. Like a near-death experience or a great loss or potentially fatal illness for an individual, collective disasters wake us up to who we are, who we can trust, what matters, and what doesn't. The difficulty is in how to stay awake when the ordinary returns.

If it does. I believe too that this pandemic is the end of something, a version of postwar prosperity for the global north predicated on exploitation of other regions, of other human beings and of nature itself, of a set of assumptions about our capacity to control that nature, of many orders that are about to become history. What arises from the ashes of this old world ending around us will be first of all a conflict as those who profit from alienation, exclusion, isolation, inequality seek to regain their footing – and as those of us who dreamed of the opposite and caught glimpses of it even in this worst of calamities seek to make something new. What all these projects around the world tell us is that they can be the foundation for bigger projects, both practically and as the imaginative and ideological basis for something new, based on generosity, abundance, horizontality, mutuality, inclusion. So what is described in this book is both practical work to meet the needs of the present and something more: the templates and maps for the future, if we are passionately committed to this vision of who else we are, if we stay awake and remember who we were at the worst of times.

Introduction

Marina Sitrin

Fear. Grief. Pain. Vulnerability. Compassion. Opening. Togetherness. Hope. Transformation …

To write or talk about this historical moment is to hold a lot of things together at once. There is a constant overarching fear, a fear that is collective and something we, people living today, have not experienced at this level of collectivity. And, while yes, we are all in the same terrible storm that is Covid-19, we are not all in the *same* boat. Structural inequality shows itself in crisis and disaster, and this one is revealing all the ugliness and systemic oppressions and inequalities most of our societies were built upon, and that privilege the very few, and try and pit the rest of us against one another.

How, then, do we function with this different individual fear and danger, and collective overarching danger? In many parts of the world we are told to fear one another, that some anonymous person is going to take our food, toilet paper or bleach. And in many cases people who could did big grocery shops, took home months' supplies of toilet paper. Why is that? Is it that we are only out for ourselves, hoarding toilet paper? Or, could it be that our fear is that the institutions of power in our societies are such that we do not believe they will take care of us – not even at the basest level – of bathroom hygiene.

There is something deep here connected to what is the real truth about who we really are, not what we are told about ourselves. Yes, we are afraid. Yes, we feel pain and vulnerability, *and* what we do with that, again and again, throughout history and now more than ever, is to reach out to one another and find ways to care for each other. We feel all of these things, and it is an and. We do not need to either fear or help, be vulnerable or open, protective or protecting, we can and are doing all of these things, and that is what makes this moment both horrific *and* transformative in a deeply hopeful way.

This book is a collection of narratives from around the world, based on interviews that took place in April of 2020. Together they give a glimpse of who we really are – the open, vulnerable, caring, brave, dedicated, compassionate and socially responsible people we are – acting with and through our collective fear. This book shines a light on aspects of our better selves, not to romanticize us, to ground us in the very real, day-to-day, ways people survive, have survived, and will continue to survive, if we listen and follow our own collective paths.

THE BOOK BECOMING

The process of this book becoming is prefigurative in many ways, as are the experiences within the chapters. Prefigurative in that it models the relationships we desire in our very acts and relationships. It began with a conversation, and then another, and another, and these expanded globally, got recorded, transcribed, translated, and within two months from inception, on Mother's Day, we collectively birthed this book. Birthing is an appropriate word here as we are mostly women, some of us already mothers.

I teach a graduate seminar on ethnography. Once the pandemic was globally apparent to us, it dominated, or was at least present, in all of our discussions. In one such conversation, in March, Seyma shared her frustration that the official government narrative in Turkey was nothing like the reality. In that case it was about people getting sick and dying, the government knowing why, yet insisting there was no virus. From there the idea germinated to look into how people around the world have been coming together in times of crisis and disaster – and find the real narrative. A small group self-selected to work on this, not as an assignment, but a labor of investigative solidarity. Seyma, Ariella, Debarati, Emre and I began.

CONTRIBUTORS AND ORGANIZATION OF THE BOOK

The contributors for this book came through friendship and political, that is, movement, networks. Ariella, Emre, Seyma and Debarati were the base from our class, then Debarati suggested Midya in Kurdistan, Northern Iraq and Chia-Hsu. Vanessa, in Brazil, who I know from Occupy Wall Street days, when she was in New York, suggested Lais, who then invited Raquel, who in turn suggested Boaventura in Mozambique. Emre, having spent time in Rojava, invited Khabat, who is based there. magalí had spoken in our class a few weeks earlier on her work in Latin America, and suggested Nancy, from Argentina. I know Liz and Eleanor from movement work over the years, EP and TP are close friends and movement participants in Greece. Neil was suggested by Ana, an Argentine in the UK. Carla, who lives on Tsleil-Waututh, Squamish, and Musqueam Lands (Vancouver, BC), I have never met in person, though we have collaborated in different movement/writing ways. Ji Young, from South Korea, was recommended by Byeong-Gwon, who in turn was suggested by Sabu, both of whom I know from anti-G8 work in Japan. This beautiful fabric of collaborators is woven of friendship and movement, the base of which guided the creation of this book.

The regions of the world discussed in this book were intentionally selected, and the countries more or less so. It was in part based on who knew someone who might want to do this, and could, in such a short time. Decisions were never based on where there was known solidarity groups and networks, as I assumed they are everywhere. And they are. There has not been a proper study yet, but from those who work in this area, the sense is that this is the largest, most diverse, mobilization of people – regular people – helping one another, under capitalism, that has ever happened.

There is a lot of privilege tied into this process, including those of us who had that bit of extra time to work on it, something many if not most people do not have – and here I am talking about clock time, as well as emotional time. The sort of privilege that allows time out to interview people, transcribe and translate those interviews, and then painfully edit the total to 3,400 words, all within a month or two, is huge. Regions of the world with intense and ongoing histories of colonialism and inequality, such as Africa, Central America and northern South America, made it harder for participants to collaborate. I want to recognize those people who wanted to participate and then, due to the violence of capitalism and the pandemic, were unable.

BORDERS AND VIOLENCE

We had a number of conversations about borders and countries, and the violence implicit in both. Had there been more time we might have organized the book thematically, to include the many areas interviewees covered, such as: prisoners' self-activity and solidarity; food production and distribution; disability self-organization and solidarity; art, music and poetry; public displays of care; mask and protection making; healthcare and self-organized health; First Nations and Indigenous organizing; education, students and teachers; pet care and animals. However, we decided that it was best to get the book in people's hands as quickly as possible, so it is organized by artificial separations, made by the dominant countries of the time for reasons of power. None of us are comfortable with this. To that end, we decided to decenter the dominating countries and, thus, Europe and North America are close to the end. Turtle Island is the landmass we have been told is North America, and that regional chapter explains the reasons, through interviews with First Nation communities and networks. It is only for reasons of space that I am not listing every group or individual interviewed in this book here, as there are close to 100. It also would not facilitate your hearing them, so please, as you read, listen carefully to the vast diversity of voices and experiences, as well as feel the commonalities.

The book begins with Rojava. I had thought to end with it, as it is the only region in this book, and with the exception of the Zapatistas in Chiapas Mexico, of the world, that is actually self-determined, self-organized and autonomous. It is not perfect, as nothing is, and really, what would that even mean if one views everything as a process and transformation? It is, however, the closest thing to a democracy in the book, a real democracy, where the people collectively make decisions about their day-to-day lives, and women are structurally as well as relationally not only equal, but have more say over things related to women. The chapter speaks for itself. The reason it is first is to begin with what is possible, on a larger scale, so that as we read all the inspiring accounts in these pages, we hold in our imaginations a possibility that is concrete and existing. It is grounding us in the possible transformation of the world, bit by bit, step by step.

PREFIGURATIVE COLLECTIVE

I don't know if it was the stories that we were facilitating, the crisis opening our hearts to more compassion, our urgent desire for a new world, that we are mostly women or/and some combination of all of these, but the result has been the most beautiful and supportive collaboration I could have imagined. Nancy wrote at one point that this project was like a life vest, and many echoed the sentiment. People volunteered to read and edit one another's chapters, countless conversations took place outside of our weekly face-to-face (computer mitigated) discussions, with those with more experience conducting interviews guiding those who had not. Writing sessions happened via computer in vastly different time zones, chapters were co-authored by people who had never collaborated and, in one case, who never had met. And the result is friendships, deep care and support, and a powerful collection of stories of solidarity and mutual aid. In two months, from beginning to end, the project was completed. This includes people working in their second and third languages.

Authorship is complicated, and often not honest in that it never fully acknowledges all the people behind a given thought, process or theory. This book is no different. As our group quickly became a collective, in many more ways than expressed above, it became clear that the book itself is a collective project. I still take responsibility for mistakes and errors, but cannot take credit for this book. We began a version of this conversation with the group, and ultimately decided to give ourselves a collective name to recognize the deeply respectful collective process. We did not have much time, and not everyone was thrilled, but we all felt good enough that we are able – and I include myself, Colectiva Sembrar – to sow seeds as a collective (in the feminine in Spanish). Had we decided to delay the book further, I would hope that these words I am writing now would have been a collective process of writing and would look different.

LANGUAGE AND POWER

On language and translation. Chia-Hsu and Nancy opened an important conversation on the power of language, and in particular dominant languages, and what is then lost in translation – not only that concepts and words are translated – but translated into dominant languages that are often those of the oppressor. As Nancy, a professional translator from Argentina, and movement participant reflected,

> Our mother tongue is, as the Russians call it, our Dearest Tongue. We know that translation, inextricably tied to geopolitical power relations, can be a double-edged sword – a tool for counter-hegemonic practices of communication and a tool of oppression, always giving minority languages a modicum of "value" in the market of linguistic exchanges.
>
> But perhaps it is key to remember here that we do not translate words. We translate ideas. And because ideas and praxes of resistance are translatable, we blandish this sword, as imperfect as our world, to cut through and reach out to those who are already building now, in their dearest tongues, a more livable world, the future we seek to imagine: precisely for that reason, their words are our words.

Please hold this in your heart and mind as you read. Some of the translations are intentionally left at what would appear, at first glance, slightly imperfect. However, listen more closely with your whole body and you can then better hear the person and place from which the author is speaking.

THE OUTWARD SPIRAL

The stories in this collection, in different ways, manifest the sort of society we could have and, in fact, already have. Our invitation with these pages is for you, our dear readers, to garner some inspiration together with concrete ideas for how to engage and expand the project that exists. This pandemic is creating small and large fissures, what we do with these openings is up to us. The new world is already being created, it is up to us to expand this creation, continuing to spiral outwards until … and then more.

About *Colectiva Sembrar*

What began as a conversation amongst a few people rapidly became a larger conversation, then a project, and naturally and beautifully a full collaboration, and birthing of a book. We, Colectiva Sembrar, are now a collective of almost all women, from around the world, dedicated to facilitating voices of those less heard who are themselves collectively creating a new society in their actions of solidarity, care, love and mutual aid. In helping to raise up these voices, we also raise our own, and yours. We see this as a very small part of many large and small projects, all acts of sowing seeds. It is up to all of us to nurture them as they grow. We, Colectiva Sembrar, are continuing this project with a website, bringing more attention to the voices in these pages, while also increasing it to include many more, in an expanding spiral of care and solidarity that we hope will reflect, suggest and transform.

PART I

Greater Middle East
(Rojava, Turkey and Iraq)

CHAPTER ONE

Communal Lifeboat: Direct Democracy in Rojava (NE Syria)

Emre Sahin and Khabat Abbas

The Autonomous Administration of North and East Syria (AANES) made international headlines for the first time during the war of Kobane against Islamic State (ISIS, DAESH) in October 2014. This global interest has been mostly militaristic. However, the remarkable and unique bottom-up political organization has created a lifeline for the peoples of North and East Syria. The Covid-19 pandemic, which is just one of several life and death crises in the region, including war and embargo, throws the AANES' bottom-up model of direct democracy into the spotlight. In this chapter, we illustrate how peoples' access to decision-making processes through communes and councils has saved lives in AANES in the current epidemic and more.

In the summer of 2012, the many different ethnic and religious communities of NE Syria joined forces to establish a pluralist, decentralized, gender-egalitarian and ecologist system of self-governance. Street communes form the base unit of this model and are represented in higher-level neighborhood or village, district and national councils. The spokespeople of the lower levels make up the members of the higher levels in this four-layered network of governance. Most social, political and economic decisions are made through the formal debates that take place among these communes and councils. Gender quotas and the co-presidency principle at all levels ensure women's equal access to decision-making processes. This governance system links communes and councils with municipalities, inspired by Kurdistan Workers' Party (PKK) leader Abdullah Öcalan's paradigm of Democratic Confederalism. In his book with the same title, Öcalan describes Democratic Confederalism as:

> This kind of rule or administration can be called a non-state political administration or a democracy without a state … States only administrate while democracies govern. States are founded on power; democracies are based on collective consensus ... Democratic confederalism … is flexible, multi-cultural, anti-monopolistic, and consensus-oriented.[1]

Surrounded by hostile neighboring states, the AANES has continuously had to be self-reliant with thousands of street communes and hundreds of neighborhood/ village and district councils working closely together to make sure basic human needs are satisfied. Shelter, food, healthcare, education and employment are not left to the mercy of the market or the state. Family-based, local and regional networks of mutual aid and solidarity ensure that nobody is homeless or starving. It is nearly impossible to find people sleeping on the street or begging for food or money in NE Syria! There are no orphanages, nursing homes or homeless shelters in the region because vulnerable members of society are not left behind. Such institutions have unfortunately become necessary across the world today due to the lack of sufficient communal care for those that need it the most urgently. Communities' direct involvement in decision-making processes in NE Syria increases their political agency and enables them to act outside the boundaries of capitalist social relations based on self-interest and competition. The gradual de-commodification of life in the region brings people together and increases their collective capability of self-sustenance. The AANES' dual system of local governance ensures peoples' access to decision-making processes and serves as a lifeboat for the communities in NE Syria at times of natural and human-made disasters. As several of our interviewees describe below, the close collaboration of communes, councils and municipalities also saved lives during the Turkish state's occupation of Serekaniye and Gire Spi in 2019.

How then has solidarity looked during the first months of the Covid-19 pandemic in a self-governed territory with collectivized and decentralized decision-making? Nation-states are often hostile to solidarity and mutual aid efforts because their existence alone exposes state failures in social welfare. What happens when, as the Zapatista saying goes, "people rule and the state obeys?"

During the early days of the pandemic, the AANES established a Central Crisis Committee bringing together representatives from the areas of education, security, health and local governance. The organization of this emergency committee reflects general political mobilization in North and East Syria, where communes and councils at all levels have representatives from the same areas responsible for policy formation and implementation. The Central Crisis Committee works in conjunction with regional committees from the seven administrative parts of Jazeera, Euphrates, Afrin, Raqqa, Tabqa, Manbij and Deir ez Zor. As co-authors of this chapter, we made five phone-interviews in April 2020 with people actively involved in solidarity, mutual aid and relief efforts in Qamishlo, NE Syria. We made an explicit effort to include voices from different levels of local governance, genders, ethnicities and ages. Like the AANES, our interviewees organize their response to the Covid-19 pandemic along the themes of local governance, health, education and security. We decided to organize the rest of this chapter similarly in order to amplify the voices of our interviewees, to whom we are thankful for inspiring us after the initial shock of the pandemic and collective inaction.

LOCAL GOVERNANCE: COMMUNES AND COUNCILS

Members of street communes and higher-level councils have stopped their regular meetings as a preventive measure to the Covid-19 pandemic. However, they have been the driving force of aid distribution efforts in NE Syria. They register the names of their neighbors that require urgent assistance, distribute food and fuel oil, and sterilize public spaces and utilities.

Heval Hikmet is a neighborhood organizer, cooperative member and computer programmer based in Qamishlo with a hopeful yet cautious account of ongoing Covid-19 efforts underlining society's high level of organization as its main strength.

Hikmet: Due to the ongoing war, embargo, and lack of health infrastructure, the current strategy here is to prevent the spread of infection and prioritize public health over the economy. We know our strengths and weaknesses, and plan accordingly. There aren't enough testing kits and ICU units, so initiatives are launched to address these issues. The health ministry is working with a Swedish institute on the development of a new test kit to produce accurate results in less than a minute. A new hospital was built in Heseke recently for corona patients only.

Our main strength is that the society is organized and public health is not less important than the economy! You are currently in the US, no? How much would they charge you if you received intensive care for corona there? Not a single dime here! With an organized society, it is easier to implement lockdown measures and make sure nobody gets left behind. There are food and oil distribution campaigns organized by the municipality to help the people in urgent need. Communes and councils have stopped their regular meetings in order to prevent spread of infection but are working remotely in coordination with municipal and other officials.

I recently finished programming a database interface to be used in hospitals across the region. With this program, all health professionals in Rojava (West Kurdistan) will have access to patient records and histories in a secure way. I started working on the database interface before the outbreak but I believe it will be useful in containment efforts. Honestly, more people are concerned about the threat of Turkish invasion than the corona pandemic itself! People are used to quarantine-type conditions because they have been living under conditions of war and embargo for almost a decade now. However, the Turkish state began its invasion with Afrin, continued with Serekaniye and Gire Spi, and poses an imminent threat to the rest of the region. We suspect a large scale Turkish state attack on Bashur (South Kurdistan) this summer.

LOCAL GOVERNANCE: MUNICIPALITIES

Municipalities are the other pillar of the AANES' dual system of local governance and have been the organizational force behind all aid distribution efforts in NE Syria. They work in close collaboration with communes and councils to deliver assistance to vulnerable groups. For example, Qamishlo Municipality is currently collaborating with a local women's clothing cooperative that has agreed to produce only face masks until the end of the pandemic. The municipality then takes these masks and delivers them to neighborhood and district council members, who have so far distributed than 40,000 masks in the city of Qamishlo.

Sharmin Shako works at Qamishlo Municipality and is playing a key role in the coordination of municipal and communal relief efforts in Qamishlo, the most densely populated part of North and East Syria.

Shako: I am a member of Qamishlo's municipal committee, which brings together 37 local municipalities in and around the city. When the corona pandemic started, we as the municipality did not stop our work and continued to address the needs of our people. We established a sterilization committee in coordination with health workers and launched a disinfection campaign to clean and sterilize all public spaces. We then converted a women's cooperative to a face-mask production workshop and have been distributing the masks made here to frontline workers to support them. We played an active role in raising awareness about the pandemic and distributed information, particularly through social media and pamphlets.

Communes are the base unit of the political system that we have been building here, and as municipalities we coordinate the efforts to respond to the peoples' needs by collaborating with communes and councils closely and in a circular way. Communes are made up of local residents who mobilize their neighbors and collect information on their specific needs and demands. Commune members then communicate these issues to neighborhood and district councils as well as our municipal committee. Policy decisions are made through the feedback that circulates among all these different groups. For example, there are municipal subcommittees responsible for food and fuel oil assistance during the pandemic. These two subcommittees work closely with local councils, whose members identify the families in their neighborhoods that are in urgent need of assistance. Our food and fuel subcommittees use this information to deliver aid to peoples' doorsteps, and the absence of distribution centers with large crowds helps us fight the spread of the virus.

Our municipality has received several volunteer initiatives from individuals and civil society organizations over the past few weeks. Each initiative is discussed at the level of its scope and impact. Regional campaigns are coordinated at the municipal level whereas initiatives at the village and neighborhood levels are organized in local councils. For example, an NGO recently launched a regional campaign in collaboration with us to provide all municipal workers with protective equipments. At the local level, communes and bakeries distributed informative pamphlets and led our campaign to raise awareness about the epidemic.

HEALTH

Since the Covid-19 pandemic is a medical issue, all segments of society in NE Syria have been mobilized to contain the infection and improve the healthcare system. The Health Ministry recently discovered a new test kit, in partnership with Pias Institute from Sweden, that detects Covid-19 infection within 30 seconds. The health representatives of the Central Crisis Committees and regional committees have been working closely with the Kurdish Red Crescent to set up medical checkpoints all across the region. Groups of engineers have created new medical equipment and are working with health, municipal and council officials to combat the spread of the virus. Engineers in Qamishlo have designed a sterilization cabinet that measures the user's temperature via motion sensors while providing sterilization cream and spray. Several of these cabinets have been set up at the entrance to important public offices. Engineers in Haseke have manufactured a new respirator with advanced features at less than a quarter of the cost of its counterparts available on the market.

Dr. Ciwan Mistefa is a Health Official at the Central Crisis Committee and the committee's only spokesperson,

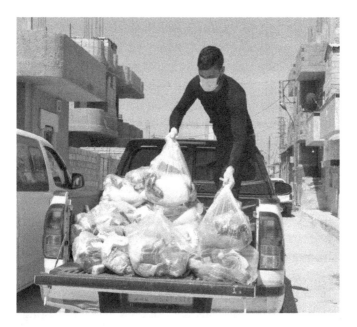

Figure 1.1 Commune collective member distributing food packets in Haseke.

reflecting the socio-political approach towards health professionals in North and East Syria during the pandemic.

Mistefa: We started taking precautionary measures
when the coronavirus spread near us in Kurdistan
Regional Government (KRG) and regime-held areas
in Syria. Our first step was to close Semelka crossing
with KRG on February 27 because corona cases were
identified there. Our main strategy was to prevent the
virus from entering here and we knew that it would
be best to take precautionary steps. Due to the war
entering its ninth year, we have limited resources in our
health sector but we took preventive steps regardless
of their cost to us. After Semelka's closure, we tight-
ened our measures and closed all border crossings,
banned gatherings, and locked down schools, markets
and other public places step by step. We stopped travel
between and within cities, set up medical points across
the region, and mobilized all our health and security
personnel and resources. This has had a big impact on
our economy, so some of these tight measures may be
loosened in future months.

I am a member of the Central Crisis Committee
of NE Syria, which we established to coordinate our
response to the coronavirus outbreak. This committee
has regional subcommittees in the seven administrative
regions, and all of these committees have representatives
from the areas of health, education, municipality, and
security. These officials are the ones actively fighting
the crisis at the frontlines. Some decisions such as the
ban on movement between cities and closing border

crossings were made by the central committee but the implementation of all decisions is done regionally as each region has specific conditions. There is constant communication and feedback among the regional and central committees. The central committee only makes decisions in response to the suggestions and debates that come from the regional committees.

Our Ministry of Health is represented in the Central Crisis Committee and has organized field teams of health professionals that report their findings and suggestions to us. As the pandemic is a medical issue, all of the decisions taken by the central committee require consultation with health workers. For example, the central committee decided to ban travel but health officials determined the details of how the ban would be implemented. Saving as many lives as possible is the goal of all of the measures we have implemented so far, and we are making sure that all corona patients in NE Syria receive their treatments without any burdens, financial or otherwise.

EDUCATION

Following the global trend, education officials in NE Syria closed down all schools and transitioned to online classes. Communes and councils played an instrumental role in this transition as they ensured the delivery of distant-education materials to students and education workers. As the default education representative of their neighborhood council, each teacher has been maintaining daily communication with their students through the WhatsApp groups they created for their classes. Groups of academics from across the world have been volunteering to give online class in their fields at Kobane and Rojava Universities.

Heval Sinan is an Education Official at the Jazeera Region Crisis Committee and has played an instrumental role in the transition to online education in the region. He emphasizes that all teachers in North and East Syria have also been education representatives of neighborhood councils, enabling close collaboration among education officials, local councils and the Ministry of Education.

> Sinan: During the debates in Jazeera Region Crisis Committee, we as educators decided to pause education at all grades on March 15 for the remainder of Spring semester because of the virus. This was not the first disruption to education here this year as the Turkish state's occupation of Serekaniye and Gri Spi last October had forced us to close schools for two months. We closed the schools near the border with Turkey because of the clashes and the schools away from the border for housing the more than 300,000 civilians that had been displaced by the invasion. This is when our online education efforts began.
>
> Our initial idea was to make up for the disruption in October and November with the use of online classes, but we decided to expand upon distant-teaching after we shut down all schools on March 15 due to the virus. Many of our students and teachers are experiencing distant-education for the first time and our transition has not been perfect. There are approximately 115,000 students in Qamishlo and some of them live in rural areas with irregular access to internet and electricity. In

close collaboration with village and street communes, we have so far identified these areas and delivered course materials in print-outs and CDs to the students and teachers living there.

Some students are struggling because they miss their friends and the classroom environment. Many teachers put in extra work to increase their familiarity with digital technologies and transform their teaching. Interestingly, these same technologies seem to have intrigued our students because their class participation has been higher than we anticipated! All of our teachers, who by the way are also education representatives in their local councils, have created WhatsApp groups for each of their classes to maintain daily communication and feedback with students. This enables us to monitor students' reception of course materials and supervise

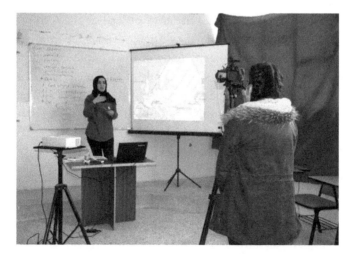

Figure 1.2   Geography teacher from Qamishlo recording her class for TV broadcast.

their transition to distant-education. I can say that more than 80 percent of our teachers and students have given us positive feedback on the transition to online classes.

SECURITY

Lastly, members of communes and councils work closely with security officials towards the implementation of lockdown measures. However, this has not been a smooth process and hundreds of civilians have been penalized for lockdown violations since March. What makes the security situation in NE Syria during the pandemic more complicated is the hostile attitude of neighboring states. The Turkish and Syrian regimes have targeted key sanitation infrastructure such as water stations, and have sabotaged the AANES' lockdown measures at borders and Qamishlo airport.

Hevi Mistefa, Internal Security official at the Central Crisis Committee, describes difficulties that the internal security forces have been facing in their implementation of lockdown measures. Thousands of ISIS members and their families continue to pose a threat to the world. She calls for international support for their detention camps.

Mistefa: Last month, we took early precautions as we closed border crossings and banned transportation between cities. We then declared curfews to limit movement within cities and implemented all these measures before the detection of any patients in the region. Our internal security personnel, 35000 in total, are working hard to implement lockdown measures and protect peoples' lives. We have been giving our members awareness training on how to avoid violent escalations during lockdown implementation.

One difficulty we face in efforts to keep infection out is the smuggling that takes place across the long border we have here. Preventing cross-border smuggling of goods and people has become more difficult during the pandemic as our forces have the double task of implementing lockdown measures within cities, prisons and camps. The Turkish and Syrian states take advantage of this situation and use the pandemic as a political tool to undermine the autonomous administration here. This is why they cut off the water to Heseke in Turkish-occupied Serekaniye. This is why they attempted to smuggle people through the regime-operated Qamishlo airport.

The burden on our shoulders has gotten worse due to the lack of international support for the maintenance of prisons and camps where we keep thousands of ISIS members and their families, many of whom are foreign nationals. We have seen multiple riots and mass-escape attempts in these prisons recently, and our forces maintain control and keep the world safe with no assistance from the detainees' countries of citizenship. To make things worse, the recent termination of the already insufficient World Health Organization relief efforts in North and East Syria is putting the lives of the five million people at stake here.

NOTE

1. Abdullah Öcalan. 2011. *Democratic Confederalism*, London: Transmedia Publishing, p. 25.

CHAPTER TWO

"Capitalism Kills, Solidarity Gives Life": A Glimpse of Solidarity Networks from Turkey

Seyma Özdemir

Mainstream media headlines in Turkey:

> COVID-19 recoveries exceed new cases as Turkey ponders normalization[1] (*Daily Sabah*)

> Turkey sends aid to nearly 30 countries in fight against Covid-19[2] (*TRT World*)

> Directorate of Communications shares a post "We are Self-Sufficient, Turkey"[3]

> Interior Minister Süleyman Soylu resigns over curfew announcement[4] (*Daily Sabah*)

> Turkey: Erdogan rejects interior minister's resignation[5] (Anadolu Agency)

Officially the Covid-19 pandemic seemed to hit Turkey late and was not discussed publicly until the first formal declaration of the first positive case. Yet, the death toll rose abruptly from the first positive case confirmed by the Minister of Health on March 11, 2020. As of May 1, the government reported 122,392 cases and 3,258 deaths. These were the tip of the iceberg, with health officials pointing out the inaccuracy of official numbers immediately silenced, often times brutally with arrests, detentions, threats.[6]

Hidden by official narratives in mainstream media, and inaudible in authoritarian discourses is the story of solidarity networks that blossomed before the outbreak was officially announced. The words of these participants are confident, their voices louder than officials' narratives The first seeds were sown in the Kadıköy and Besiktas districts of Istanbul. They have been flourishing ever since. Today solidarity networks operate in 15 districts – Ataşehir, Avcılar, Bahçelievler, Beşiktaş, Esat, Kadıköy, Kartal, Maltepe, Mersin, Nurtepe-Güzeltepe, Sancaktepe, Sarıyer, Şişli, Tuzluçayır, Zeytinburnu,[7] and in the provinces of Bursa and Ayvalık (Balıkesir).

From food delivery to legal help, from women's autonomous collectives to educational support, solidarity networks have built "a paradise in the hell" in Turkey.[8] Volunteers from Ataşehir, Kadıköy, Beşiktaş, Çekmeköy and Ayvalık[9] generously and immediately agreed to share stories as print interviews upon my contacting them. They insisted on collective responses, writing "we"; that is, how they make decisions and act. My interviews focused on their experiences; whether their relationships and new ways of doing things might last through and beyond the crisis; on the different feelings of people; and their imaginings of the post-crisis.

This chapter glimpses Turkey's solidarity networks. Discussed first is the context of Turkey through the eyes of solidarity networks, then their mobilization, their encounters, and concluding with remarks on re-imagined and unimagined spaces.

Loyal to their insistence on first-person plurality and collective agency, the interviewees use the local collectives' district and province names. These networks represent more than a hundred volunteers,[10] telling us a momentous story amidst pressure from "official" accounts to silence what they say, obscure what they do and befog what they imagine.

CONTEXT THROUGH THE EYES OF SOLIDARITY NETWORKS

Recep Tayyip Erdogan (president of Turkey) declared a Coronavirus Relief Package in which the resources of the state were allocated to the employers, business owners, with nothing for the people except for cologne and

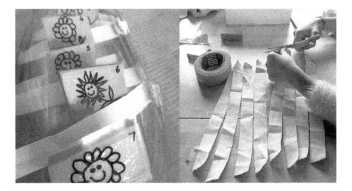

Figures 2.1 and 2.2 Neighborhood outreach material from the Kadıköy Solidarity Network. (Photos courtesy of Colectiva Sembrar)

prayers. Declared on March 18, 2020, media reported "measures to primarily relieve companies, including a six-month deferral of various taxes and social security premiums, a three-month deferral of loan repayments to public banks and other assistance for those indebted to private lenders ... The poor were promised partial increases in existing social benefits, while citizens aged over 65 had to content themselves with free masks and germ-killing traditional cologne."[11] We read this as people being left alone, struggling with this disaster. We started to discuss how to organize locally. (Kadıköy, Facebook Livestream, March 26, 2020)

We got the message that everyone should take care of themselves. We continued to do what we know best – expanding our solidarity networks. So, "everyone should stay home" but if 90 percent of the population are not ones who will stay at home, who is the nation? While recommending staying at home, they continued building Canal Istanbul ["championed by President Tayyip Erdogan" but "criticized by opponents for its negative environmental impact"[12]]. This is insane. (Kadıköy, Facebook Livestream, March 26, 2020)

When we look at the current government, we can see how strange they find the situation. We saw the inefficiency of other institutions and saw that what the government was doing was not enough. People must take fate into their hands, must create solutions themselves. We want to create a solidarity culture. (Beşiktaş, Facebook Livestream, April 19, 2020)

This government saw the "danger" of solidarity networks and the Ministry of Interior Affairs immediately announced that "No one can help other than us. It is forbidden!" [The Interior Ministry instructed all governor's offices not to collect financial aid unless the provincial governor allowed it.[13]] Capitalist modernity would like to obscure any sort of solidarity webs to maintain culture submissiveness. This is a great opportunity in two ways: what really matters is not the state, it is the people living together. Secondly, people can claim agency and have the power to create solutions to their problems without a state, a governing power above, of course in a local level.

We say that another world is possible, so we are now building that political culture, the prototypes of that possibility in this process of pandemic. This is a historical moment. It is a moment that demonstrates the inability of governing. This is actually becoming an agent. This exists in our culture but the system pushes you to forget it, the system tells you that we will give you orders, what to do and how to do it. If there is any problem, you won't raise your voice and question so much, and you won't dare to search for solutions with the ones around you. But now people remember that, well, this is what a society is, this is what we were before.

We know that this particular government and any system based on the marriage of capital and the state will not do any good for laborers. This pandemic showed this very clearly. Campaigns of "Stay Home" did not consider the brutal conditions laborers work in. Even the new legislative measures show that this pandemic benefits employers and pushes laborers into the margins of extreme poverty. (Ataşehir, Interview, April 4, 2020)

All we have done illustrates all the problems of the system, the government, its incompetence, and their intentions and unwillingness to take care of people. The things done by a bunch of volunteers shows those who cannot be handled by destructive states. Although various NGOs, the government and municipalities deliver assistance, we know that these assistance programs are not adequate since the government billed this crisis to the essential workers. (Fatih, Interview, April 4, 2020)

GETTING ORGANIZED: FROM LOCAL COUNCILS TO RE-IMAGINED AND UNIMAGINED SPACES

We know each other from various democratic organizations, workers' unions, collectives, and various political groups in Kadıköy. We contacted each other, got organized very fast and announced Kadıköy Solidarity Network within four days of the Ministry of Health acknowledging the first positive case. First, we created a private Facebook group and invited people we know and trust. Our numbers grew very fast. We prepared posters and shared three phone numbers and stated that we are ready to help our neighbors over 65 with chronic disease [on whom the government imposed a curfew, March 21]. All this happened in a couple of days.

Then we created an online application to volunteer: including questions such as what potentials/resources they have [to share], in which neighborhood they reside, and what they can do with solidarity networks. The number of volunteers grew. Many people submitted applications. Every single day it increased even more. As the organizers of the networks, we are in contact with each other day and night. We call each other, text each other. We use different applications such as WhatsApp, and Telegram but of course they are not enough. We occasionally meet in person as small groups as well. (Kadıköy, Interview, April 4, 2020)

We are thinking of how to include local artisans, how we can cook for each other, as well as seed sharing to produce our own food. This is a politics of agriculture, we foresee a food crisis. Since seeds are imported, we are trying to prepare for that. This is about meeting basic needs. When this crisis is over, how can we grow our food by utilizing a tiny area between ten buildings? (Kadıköy, Facebook Livestream, April 19, 2020)

After the foundation of Kadıköy Solidarity Network, we organized a Facebook group and invited people to join us. Each of us added acquaintances from the district. This created a sort of organic link with people who rarely meet. We created social media accounts to gather volunteers and shared contacts. We hold meetings every week. In these meetings we talk about new needs, experiences, and suggestions, and plan accordingly. We made posters put on the doors of buildings in our neighborhoods. Volunteers ask their neighbors what they need in their buildings, streets and neighborhoods in order to identify basic needs. People saw the posters, and through social media learned our phone numbers.

People now share our contact information, many in the beginning without believing that this solidarity was real. We received many different calls, and tried to connect those with resources to those without. Some wanted us to help them pay their utility bills, or to get medicine for their pets. We learned that many need legal assistance. Many people suffering health problems other than coronavirus don't have the access to health care. Thus, we are organizing to supply public health facilities and legal assistance with the help of volunteers who are legal and health professionals. (Beşiktaş, Interview, April 4, 2020)

Ataşehir Solidarity Network exemplifies Kadıköy and Beşiktaş Solidarity networks. It was founded with the initiative of a bunch of friends from Örnek and Mustafa Kemal.[14] We are still taking baby steps. By the end of March we came together and started to think about how to organize solidarity networks in neighborhoods at a district level. Our first principle was to raise our voice as citizens and to solidify our solidarity networks by focusing on shared necessities. In our first meeting, we took other solidarity networks activities into consideration and discussed how to proceed in the short, middle, and longer term. Although everyone was responsible for every task, we distributed main duties such as social media management, creating images/forms, coordination of contact, gathering the supplies, finding places, and contact with other networks to organize immediately.

By the beginning of April, we created our Facebook and Twitter accounts. We added our friends and asked to add their acquaintances. We first contacted *muhtar-lıklar* [local neighborhood administration] and started to learn what had been done for our neighbors [administratively]. We realized that a lot of neighbors were not aware of support channels. We organized to deliver them supplies. We found a place to use as storage and prepare face shields and masks. We contacted the local health center and learned what they need in 1 Mayis neighborhood. Then we started making essentials for health workers, in addition to grocery shopping, looking after the pets, gathering food and cleaning essential donations from our volunteers and delivering them to people in need. (Ataşehir, Interview, April 4, 2020)

As Fatih Solidarity Network we have a history which goes back to the 2013 Gezi Park rebellion. Since then we have come together in neighborhood councils to discuss politics, including issues that pertain to our neighborhood and then present our response. For the last year, we focused on our local needs. By 2020 we gathered with young friends in our neighborhood, and began tutoring, film screenings, and organizing seminars. We channeled this collective to deal with the needs that emerged during the coronavirus pandemic.

First, we launched a campaign to reach people laid off and in urgent need. We gathered information about needs of families/household in Fatih and places close to Koca Mustafa Paşa [a critical district of Istanbul very close to one of the biggest hospitals] and organized through social media. We grocery shopped, packed and delivered to families in need. The most needed items were food and children's essentials. We learned that health workers in Koca Mustafa Pasa work under very difficult conditions and even have no food in hospitals. Volunteers started cooking for health workers, and we delivered food to them. (Fatih, Interview, April 4, 2020)

We have been organizing through Çekmeköy Solidarity network. Those who stayed at home immediately opened social media accounts and began to deliver food to high risk neighbors and acquaintances laid off. Then we started to organize legal help from our friends who are lawyers for people in need of legal assistance. We directed them to the solidarity networks of lawyers. (Çekmeköy, Interview, April 4, 2020)

Ayvalık Local Initiative formed on January 5, 2019 after the forum "What kind of a local organization/administration do we want, and how can we organize it?" by invitation from Ayvalık Democracy Platform. Forum participants, after discussing our problems and needs, decided to come up with solutions through neighborhood councils. After the forum, we announced the commencement of the Ayvalık Local Initiative. We stated that we wanted to come together with various workers' unions, women's collectives/organizations, environmental organizations, and created a social contract (at the provincial level). We invited people who reside in Ayvalık – immigrants, students, artisans – and we still welcome many volunteers. We divided volunteers into two groups; one makes face shields and masks, the other delivers this equipment to health workers at public hospitals and local health centers; postal, cargo and grocery store workers. We simultaneously produce and deliver PPEs. (Ayvalık, Interview, April 4, 2020)

ENCOUNTERS: "YOU REMINDED US THAT WE ARE HUMAN BEINGS"

As we were the first among the solidarity networks which got organized pretty fast right after the outbreak, we became widely known. We have been receiving calls from many districts and provinces … We received a call from Çankırı State Hospital [a province 468 km from Istanbul]. Doctors requested face shields, so we sent shields. Our friends who make shields wrote notes on the boxes "We love you so much! We can't be without you!" If I were a doctor, and received these masks and shields and these notes from a person very far way, whom I didn't know, when the state was not even able to provide me with surgical masks …

Solidarity makes people feel incredible emotions nowadays. My phone number is one of the contact numbers on posters. We hear this sentence many, many times: "You reminded us that we are human beings!" I heard this both from those who have resources to share and those who are in need. This is so real! Solidarity makes us human beings indeed! People calling me, especially the ones 80–90 years old, tell me that they would like to see my face when these days are over, and meet over a coffee. Yes, I reply, "We will definitely meet one day." The system, the state that you pay taxes to wants to get rid of you, leave you to death .... However, there are others who care about you, who stick by you in solidarity without any expectation. Then you start feeling like a society ... You start realizing that you are in the same boat, whether young or old, employed or unemployed, health worker, baker, as ones who have been left to their own destiny. You realize that you are stronger together and you must act collectively! (Kadıköy, Interview, April 4, 2020)

This person who called us had been deprived of almost everything. She has nothing, no food, she takes care of her grandchild but can't even afford diapers. We solved her problems with solidarity. But this is not enough. We bring her materials so she can make face shields. In solidarity, although we don't expect anything in return, everyone should feel she can contribute. Not to feel helpless, rather to see herself as expanding the scope of solidarity, to see her own power, our power and to trust herself in order to trust us. (Kadıköy, Interview, April 4, 2020)

We know we have a new collective consciousness, reset after the pandemic. We have met many neighbors who told us that they will do whatever they can since meeting us. Our mommy [a common Turkish reference to an older woman] who couldn't sew masks since she is very old, started to cut elastic for masks and she feels wonderful. (Beşiktaş, Interview, April 4, 2020)

People at first don't understand that we are doing these things without any expectations. They are used to the vertical form of interaction with the state, institutions … They can't quite understand when they hear this sort of "horizontal[15]" solidarity networks, as it is very different from vertical interaction. They ask, "why don't you ask for money?" This is a great opportunity to flourish solidarity networks. (Beşiktaş, Facebook Livestream April 19, 2020)

REINVENTION SOLIDARITY CULTURES RE-IMAGINING SPACES AND SOCIETIES: "THE KING IS NAKED!"

This is a way of asserting "The King is Naked!" or crying "Who is the state?" as our old auntie did with her rod in Cerratepe. [One of the most beautiful districts of Artvin, in Northeast Turkey, Cerratepe activists have struggled for years to stop mining there. One of the old women protestors yelled "Who is the state? If there are no people, then there is no state."] Solidarity networks show us that we should take fate into our hands, not only to show it is possible but also an obligation. We foresee if we struggle, persevere, we can succeed in everything step by step. We need to find alternative tools in this process, not to rely on capital and ruling classes. (Ayvalık, Interview, April 4, 2020)

We have a shared problem. Even though we come from different backgrounds [as volunteers] we re-learn a common language thinking together, we learn how to abandon our "selves" and start to question our boundaries, prejudices, and realize the possibilities/potentials. (Ataşehir, Interview, April 4, 2020)

We are living in a social formation and network of relations in which competition, alienation, loneliness, antagonism, relationships based on self-interest, accumulation, selfishness, have been valued, encouraged, even sanctified. Everything was there to satisfy the needs of that sacred "I" … Then we realized that we are quite similar to the people around us, even those we didn't dare touch. We imagine a society in which everyone supports each other with respect to her skills, professions, resources through solidarity networks. Now I imagine altruism, mutual aid and solidarity as thinking of the ones around you, holding hands, fellowship, and genuine/real power/force. (Beşiktaş, Interview, April 4, 2020)

Capitalism cannot solve one single problem we have, even perfunctorily. In the cases like today, the system is locked. I always think that if we as the people, laborers, will take charge we would definitely do a lot better than today in the field of education, health care, traffic, anything. Many people who did not think like this now think as such. First and foremost, people question the very existence of the state today. If it collects taxes from us, if it erases the debts of big companies at once and for all, and cannot provide the laborers with paid leaves in today's turmoil, and cannot supply basic food and health care, why does it exist? What does the state do other than show us a stick? The links the solidarity networks organize, I think these are seeds for self-organization in every neighborhood. (Kadıköy, Interview, April 4, 2020)

In this process we see how precious solidarity networks are and how fast people can organize. People feel better when they come and think together, learn together, decide collectively. We are in a learning process – to act collectively, in collaboration with each other. Our people can feel very significant agents/actors. How fast our solidarity networks grow, if people stand by not just giving charity. (Çekmeköy, Interview, April 4, 2020)

Has your best childhood friend ever moved to the city you live in years later? Mine did. It feels so wonderful. You can't remember every single thing you experienced together, but you feel enormously happy. You immediately continue where you left off. You rediscover things that you enjoy doing together. All your belongings are hers and hers are yours. You wouldn't be afraid of getting hurt for each other. You would give up privileges for each other. You would become courageous. Because she is your childhood. Even though you would lose everything, you couldn't dare hurt your childhood. You see, these are our childhood relationships – without expectations, unsparing, and the relations which should persist. We are happy when we get tired. We become childhood friends when we meet with our neighbors. We trust more when we get more exhausted. You want to make more friends, become comrades with everyone. You immediately begin to see the goodness in people. (Beşiktaş, Interview, April 4, 2020)

NOTES

1. www.dailysabah.com/turkey/covid-19-recoveries-exceed-new-cases-as-turkey-ponders-normalization/news (accessed May 19, 2020).
2. www.trtworld.com/turkey/turkey-sends-aid-to-nearly-30-countries-in-fight-against-covid-19-35290 (accessed May 19, 2020).
3. www.iletisim.gov.tr/english/haberler/detay/directorate-of-communications-shares-a-post-we-are-self-sufficient-turkey (accessed May 19, 2020).
4. www.dailysabah.com/politics/interior-minister-suleyman-soylu-resigns-over-curfew-announcement/news (accessed May 19, 2020).
5. www.aa.com.tr/en/politics/turkey-erdogan-rejects-interior-ministers-resignation/1802348 (accessed May 19, 2020).
6. https://t24.com.tr/haber/ankara-universitesi-video-goruntusu-hakkinda-inceleme-baslatildi-gerekli-uyarilar-yapildi,867333 (accessed May 19, 2020).
7. https://dayanismaagi.org/ (accessed May 19, 2020).
8. Rebecca Solnit. 2009. *A Paradise Built in Hell: The Extraordinary Communities that Arise in Disasters.* New York: Viking.
9. District of Balıkesir in Western Turkey.
10. Solidarity networks responded to written interviews and I used livestreams launched by volunteers.
11. Read more: www.al-monitor.com/pulse/originals/2020/03/turkey-coronavirus-aid-package-bring-little-relief-economy.html#ixzz6LCSTTeSt (accessed May 19, 2020).
12. www.reuters.com/article/us-turkey-canal/turkey-holds-first-tender-related-to-istanbul-canal-project-idUSKBN21D1WY (accessed May 19, 2020).
13. www.reuters.com/article/health-coronavirus-turkey-cenbank/turkish-central-bank-donates-15-million-to-turkish-coronavirus-fundraiser-idUSI7N2AX019 (accessed May 19, 2020).

14. They iterate the name of the neighborhood, 1 Mayıs (Mayday). They prefer this name, significantly because the name changed to Mustafa Kemal after the 1980 coup d'état. Mustafa Kemal (Ataturk – Father of the Turk) was the "official" founder of the Republic of Turkey after the foundation of the Republic.

15. This beautifully echoes *horizontalidad* in Marina Sitrin. 2016. *Horizontalism: Voices of Popular Power in Argentina.* Edinburgh, Scotland: AK Press.

CHAPTER THREE

Solidarity Network in Iraq During Covid-19: This Time the Enemy is Invisible

Midya Khudhur

INTRODUCTION

In the last days of February 2020, in the city of Najaf, 100 miles south of Baghdad, an Iranian student fainted, falling on the ground. Soon after, reports circulated that he had been infected with Covid-19. This was the first encounter in Iraq with the virus, and shortly after, an uneasy atmosphere prevailed over the country as reporting of confirmed cases escalated. Based on that, a lockdown was decided on March 14, 2020, for most Iraqi cities.

At the beginning of the lockdown, people were committed and collaborating with the authorities. Yet soon after many people lost their business, students in public schools were not offered online courses, domestic violence increased, salaries were not paid on time, and another stream of poverty was faced by people whose living is based on daily earnings.

The situation in Iraq was not steady even before Covid-19; the country was still recovering from the ISIS crisis.

Things were not stable as an angry uprising (the October Revolution of late 2019) had not yet fully subsided in the central and southern parts of Iraq. The demonstrations caused a high number of deaths and injuries, yet it did not stop the will of those people even after the official resignation of Prime Minster Adil Abdul-Mahdi. They want to put an end to the corruption in this country.

The northern part of Iraq, which is of Kurdish majority and ruled by the Kurdistan Regional Government (KRG), was also not politically and economically ready for such a crisis. KRG was facing an economic downturn since the attack of ISIS in 2014, accompanied by great political tension with the central government over the distribution of the budget, followed by the referendum for independence that caused severe consequences for Kurds. Furthermore, the region is host to over 1.5 million internally displaced people (IDP) and Syrian refugees. All of these factors contributed to the rise in poverty, joblessness and mistrust between people and their government.

In this chapter, I interviewed people from different geographical locations in Iraq. Rasan and Las are from Kurdistan Region of Iraq; therefore, their political context is different from Layla and Noor, who are living in the southern part of Iraq, which is ruled by the central government.

RASAN DUHOKI

Rasan is a 25-year-old humanitarian activist, from Duhok governorate in the north of the Kurdistan Region. His city has been hosting refugees and IDPs since 2011.

With the great flux of displaced people, in 2014, Rasan became an active participant in supporting his community. He joined numerous volunteer projects and initiated many of them. In 2016 he established his organization Rusaz, meaning a new face. Rasan still often prefers doing personal solidarity work, to deliver assistance to people as quickly as possible. His aim is more to provide aid than acquire a profitable professional career in the humanitarian sector. As the lockdown continued, Rasan found it urgent to support people with high needs and low access to resources.

How did you begin your solidarity efforts during this pandemic?
As the negative sides of the lockdown began to appear, I wanted to start from myself before putting the blame on anyone or the authorities. I decided to make contributions in the fastest and easiest way possible; therefore, I preferred delivering assistance by myself without carrying the name of the NGO. I began to withdraw money from my savings, and worked on creating a list of the families that I need to assist. I coordinated with a retailer, who helped me to arrange food baskets. I could reach up to 100 households in the first period. Later more people donated money and therefore the scale of the assistance increased; we offered food baskets and medications. I also coordinated with a friend of mine, who is a pharmacy owner; he donated to offer all the medications that those people needed in this period. He tries to help them as much as he can.

What is the difference between this crisis and the past ones that your community has faced?

The difference this time is that the whole world is facing this pandemic. It is not restricted to a certain country or community; all experiencing the same fear. Yet, in the past crisis, we would receive support from other countries, like the scenario was when ISIS attacked Iraq, but now, we all have to depend on ourselves, we all are in the same boat together. And what makes it difficult is that this virus has no borders, it is not only a city, a camp, or a community, it is a borderless virus. One needs to think about how to support effectively, especially that in Duhok, we do not have reliable statistics for people who are at the poverty level.

What are other collaboration stories you have heard and want to share?

I heard this story from the retailer I buy food commodities from, he told me about a businessman who made an agreement with him that he would send a group of young people to him to get food baskets for people in need. I checked the amount of money that this anonymous man has to pay and it was $90,000 in less than two months. I also heard of a member of the parliament, he has been in touch with an association for people of special needs, and has contributed an amount of money for each family and also covered their rent. This was inspiring and encouraging to me, especially that they did not use his contribution as a way to show off on social media platforms.

Are there things that you discovered about yourself in the period of the lockdown?

Yes, in the past, I would drive the car for something that was a 10-minute walking distance, just to get bread and groceries for my family, but now, I am doing those basic things by walking. I think I discovered that I should walk more when it comes to things that can be accessed without the use of the car. I also learned that I could spend days without going to restaurants and cafes. Before the lockdown, I would go at least twice a day to those places, which is unnecessary and unhealthy.

What surprised you and inspired you the most?

The coordination between the government and the people was so inspiring. The region is already going

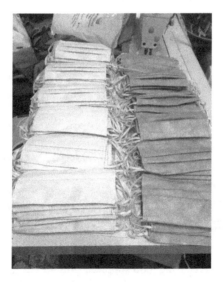

Figure 3.1   Making masks, Samawah.
(Photo courtesy of Layla Ali)

through a hard time due to the general political and economic scenario in Iraq, but it managed this situation very well. This time we felt that we are taken care of, I think the government made smart plans to respond to this crisis.

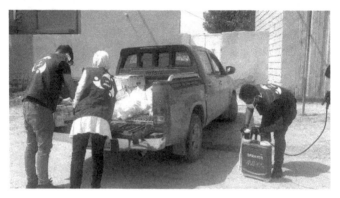

Figure 3.2   Preparing food supplies, Samawah. Rasan giving masks to police officers. (Photo courtesy of Layla Ali)

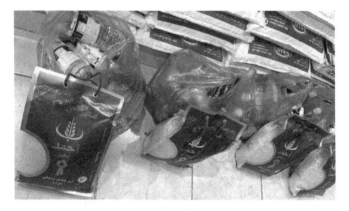

Figure 3.3   Preparing food supplies, Duhok. The dry food is a sample of what Rasan has donated. (Photo courtesy of Rasan Duhoki)

LAS RASHEED

Las is a 30-year-old humanitarian worker, from the city of Sulaymaniyah in East Kurdistan, but he stays in Erbil, the capital of the Kurdistan Region, for work. As the KRG announced the lockdown, Las decided to return to his city to spend this period with his family instead of staying all alone in his apartment in Erbil.

How is the pandemic affecting you? How does your country/city manage it?
The authorities made strict measures to minimize the harm because of corona and people, so far, have shown respect to the regulations. It is actually surprising that this is the first time in 20 years KRG and people are working in harmony! As for me, I am continuing my work routine, yet from home. I am trying to enjoy spending time with my family, reading, or video gaming; therefore, I do not think the pandemic has got me bored of the lockdown as I have many resources.

How has the situation affected people around you? How are you helping each other in this tough period?
I live at the center of Sulaymaniyah, I have many people in my neighborhood whose source of income depends on their daily labor, but as there is a lockdown, they are not allowed to work. Therefore, many of us try to get in touch with vulnerable people either via our connections or through social media. My mother and brother are regularly obtaining medications for an old lady who lives 5 minutes away from us. I also know our neighbor next door is buying food to another older lady living on

the block behind us. Even though I am directly involved in this pandemic response on a professional level, I feel I am also playing a good role in finding people in need and directing them to people who can support them. I am also helping a friend of mine who is fostering a dog from a shelter by providing dog food. Despite all of this, I think the least thing that myself or any of us can do is being committed to the regulations provided by the health department.

What has inspired you the most in this period?
What makes me happy and proud the most is seeing people giving attention to stray animals and providing them with food. Three of my friends are collecting bones and meat for those animals. This would never be the scenario ten years ago, no one would care about animals, but it is happening now. This work is done by normal people, not by an NGO or local authorities. It means that our people realize some matters can be handled by themselves instead of relying on the government only. It's always heartwarming and reassuring to see that in a war-torn region, humanity and kindness still prevails.

Any last thoughts you want to add?
This pandemic was not expected, but our region has already been through many crises, and this has taught people resilience. The first few days were full of panic, people were rushing to food markets buying large quantities of supplies, but that did not last more than a few days. People knew that this is not the end of the world, and there will always be a way to survive since we know

from experience, as we had food scarcity in the 90s of the last century. For instance, food markets decide not to sell more than two bags of rice to the same person, since others will need it too. This again showed how common interest prevailed, and short term gains in businesses were put aside. I witnessed this every weekend when I went to buy my household's daily needs.

NOOR AL-TAAI

Noor is a university professor in her early 30s. She lives in Basrah in the Southeast of Iraq and has recently moved to a new apartment with her partner as she is a newly wedded bride. Due to the outbreak, Noor and her husband spent their honeymoon in lockdown in their apartment. The pandemic hit Noor on a personal and professional level. She had great concerns about how to adopt the new online learning system and how to make it workable for her students. She is worried about her students losing an academic year, as they have already missed many classes because of the demonstrations in Iraq that started earlier in October 2019.

How were your first encounters with Covid-19?
In the beginning, when the news was spreading that corona is emerging in Iraq, people did not think it can be a serious and deadly virus. I thought that the lockdown is only a short and temporary state; therefore, I thought that it is a good opportunity for me to have a rest and do things I have always been putting off, yet soon anxiety took its part. I started to get worried about

my mother, as she has eczema. I stopped visiting her fearing that I may harm her or transfer the virus to her. Anxiety shortly increased, and I was afraid and terrified of everything. One day I wanted to have a walk outside, I could not make it more than a few steps, I felt that everything around me is carrying the virus, even the air; I soon went inside because my apartment is the safest place I could be at.

How did online teaching effect you?
When the Ministry of Education decided to change learning into an online system, my concerns shifted from my protection into how I can conduct my lessons in the best way to students, especially that I have up to 500 students per one class. This is challenging, as the internet service is not good in Iraq, and we do not have great technology resources. I, with other teachers, we needed to search and explore new tools that the virtual world offers to conduct our lessons.

Was there something notable in academia in this period?
Yes, a professor at the University of Basrah worked on developing a solution that can detect if someone is infected with the corona faster than the one we have exported from outside. His invention was successful, and his solution was sent out to the other governorate as well. This is brilliant and shows a positive side of the pandemic.

How is your community showing solidarity in this period?
Our neighbor is a religious figure; he heard of a fatwa that everyone should donate money for those who are in need. Therefore, he decided to collect money from

people who live in our building and buy food baskets, and so he collected money from us too. I felt so happy, yet I was also worried about the families that we could not reach to support. I also heard about a senior student in our university who bought gloves and face masks to give them to the security forces. He did this from his budget.

What are the current social issues you want to highlight?
Here it is becoming a problem how to deal with the corpses that are carrying the virus; people are afraid to follow the Islamic regulations to wash the corpse and bury it. I have heard a story of a man who died because of corona and his family refused to receive his corpse and bury him. Not all the cemeteries are allowing having bodies with corona in their place. The only way for this corpse to be buried was when someone from Hashd al-Shaabi volunteered to bury the body himself, believing that it is a religious duty and the power of God is greater than the power of a virus.

Corona is also imposing new social traditions. As you know, when we women greet each other we also kiss each other's cheeks. The other day I went to a nurse in my neighborhood for medications, she came to hug me but I pushed her away, it was not appropriate and I made her feel awkward, but we have to be protective. Moreover, unfortunately, some people are looking down to those who are having positive results for the corona, families are feeling ashamed to reveal if one of their member is infected.

LAYLA ALI

Layla is a single mom in her 40s and a humanitarian worker who served for 23 years in this sector in Iraq. She lives in the city of Samawah (175 miles southeast of Baghdad) with her daughter and mother. For her work, she needs to constantly travel to Baghdad and stay there during the week, yet she was in Samawah and on leave during the time the Iraqi government announced the lockdown. Therefore, she has now been with her family for more than two months, working from home and managing the household responsibilities.

How does your community perceive Covid-19?
I think Iraq holds a very different status in its perseverance against the virus. Social solidarity in Iraq existed since long ago before the pandemic. People think that it is a religious duty and a humanitarian feeling that they must have toward each other. Iraq has always been through hard times, starting from its history of wars during Saddam's time, and the post-American invasion where the sectarian war increased among the Iraqis and the clash of power in our government. Iraqis in recent years have been through a lot of suffering, and it is just starting to recover from the harm that ISIS has done to our country. Therefore, with this entire unsteady situation, the amount of poverty and insecurity increased in Iraq. Nevertheless, social coherence and solidarity have always been there among the Iraqi people, and eventually, their reaction to the coronavirus was less panicked than other countries.

Can you explain further the forms of social collaboration in your community?

I think we are lucky to have the Iraqi younger generation (born in the 1990s and later) active and ready to dedicate their energy to support our community. I personally have been in contact with a group of young people for years, and make my donations through them, as they can better locate people who require support. I am used to giving away money for donation each month, even before the pandemic, I also take care of two orphans that I have never met, I only know them through photos. I continuously provide them with monthly cash assistance until they become adults, then I shift my donations to another group of orphans.

During this pandemic, did your assistance take a new form?

Yes, in this crisis, my daughter and I have increased the usual amount of money that we donate per month. We give them to the same group of people, and on their behalf, instead of only offering food supplies, they have also added cleaning and medical supplies to the baskets they are distributing. Our donations also go to a group of females who have volunteered to buy cloth and make masks for free. Some of those ladies are already tailors, and some of them do it as a hobby. Those masks are made for people in the health sector, the security forces who are spending the whole day on the street to prevent any sort of gatherings, and they also give them to normal people on the street who are not wearing masks.

Are there other activities by people around you that you want to share?

The Iraqi government offered to provide a grant for those people who require financial support, and as you know, most of those people live in a poor and rural area. Many of them are illiterate or do not have appropriate access to the internet. I know some people spread the news that they are ready to fill out the applications for those people for free and help them to apply for the grant. Young people around me are trying their best to support us and raise solidarity. I also know another group that offers printed copies with instructions on how to protect oneself from the virus. They distribute those flyers to a high number of families.

I think such initiatives are very important; we have to support our community. We should not have people suffering from hunger. Otherwise, they would never care if they die because of the virus.

Any last thoughts you want to add?

This time the experience of Iraq is different; for many people, this pandemic is more bearable than many other things that have happened in the past. This time our enemy is hidden, not like it has been, it is not a sectarian war, not ISIS, and not the government. Everyone is equal now, the virus does not differentiate you according to your race and ethnicity, and it can kill a leader as well as a poor boy. This time Iraq is not standing alone in a crisis; it is a universal issue. This pandemic united all the Iraqis, just like when we watch a football match, and all the Iraqis, with its different races, support the Iraqi team. We get so happy when we know a city is overcoming corona. It is a lesson to humanity that we all are of very little power compared to the power of God. We should learn to stop living like we are in a forest. We do not have to kill each other to live; there is space for all of us to have a share of this life. A tiny creature can kill us all and deprive us of saying goodbye to our loved ones. We have to know that we all are equal, and nothing lasts forever. We have to make the best out of what we have.

PART II

South and East Asia
(Taiwan, South Korea and India)

CHAPTER FOUR

Sharing Spaces and Crossing Borders: Voices from Taiwan

Chia-Hsu Jessica Chang

In the modern/colonial world, we are disciplined to be lonely. The oppressors call this loneliness "individuality." They try and make us believe that the body of an ideal individual is impermeable and intact. Therefore, we imagine the impermeable and intact spaces to safely contain our bodies, and we reify such spaces by cutting through places with racial, gender, and national borders. We are made to believe that we cannot share space with others. We are trained to be untrusting of our people and our loved ones. Places are torn apart into segregated fragments, so are our collective body and collective self. We are lonely, indeed, because reaching across each other's pain, deaths, desires and love became difficult.

But we resist. We experiment. Many people around the world are with us. We know that bordered spaces and individualized bodies are violent designs. We undo borders and create shared spaces. We not only acknowledge but also actively embrace our bodies' vulnerability and permeability. In the midst of a pandemic, shared spaces and permeable bodies should not increase our fear as the oppressors tell us, but instead should be our survival kit. A web of communal support with strategic physical distancing does not equate to social segregation.

In this chapter, I bring together six collective voices from Taiwan to think about shared spaces. Many international media outlets have been praising the Taiwanese state for its successful Covid-19 prevention. Very few local people's daily practices and knowledge are visible in the global vision. I suggest that local people's practices and knowledge are at the core of the Covid-19 prevention which the state cannot do without. While the following six collective voices may all come from Taiwan, they do not monopolize the representation of Taiwanese; they also do not speak for each other. I bring them together in conversation, not in comparison or in competition.

Let's keep in mind that we are using a colonial language to strategically build a coalition with people who do not use English in their daily life or do not speak it at all. Some meanings might be lost or transculturated in my translation or in our reading process. In this language and cultural power dynamic, I hope we are vulnerable, permeable and ready to weave new relations.

COMMUNAL PRACTICES AND LOCAL KNOWLEDGES IN PLACES

In order to claim a space back from an oppressive design, we need to see the space as inseparable from its dwellers. We need to see the communal practices that the dwellers do based on their localized knowledge. We need to listen to their logics.

Hsin-Kang

Far away from metropolitan cities, Hsin-Kang Township is located in Jiayi County in Southern Taiwan, the county with the most aged population in Taiwan. While the official household record shows that the elderly represent over 20 percent of the total population, the reality is that the elderly represent 50 percent of the total population due to the severe outflow of the younger populations. Many young adults have to work in bigger towns or cities to financially sustain their families in Hsin-Kang, and, as a result, leave their children in Hsin-Kang to stay with grandparents. Therefore, in addition to the single-elder or duo-elder families, there are many grandparent-rearing families in Hsin-Kang. Besides, a good number of immigrant spouses from Southeast Asia and China settle in Hsin-Kang but struggle to become an organic part of the township.

Chin-Huang Chen offers insight into how Hsin-Kang residents live a sustainable communal life and tackle Covid-19. Chen is a dedicated local doctor, born and raised in Hsin-Kang. He attended medical school in Taipei in 1970 and returned to his hometown in 1981. In 1987, the Dajiale Lottery[1] (translation: Fun For All Lottery) and sexualized performances on the electric flower cars[2] were popular in Hsin-Kang. Chen realized that the gambling and sexist visual cultures were harmful to Hsin-Kang residents' psychology, but he could not do much about it in his clinic. Therefore, initiated by a donation from Hwai-Ming Lin (the leader and choreographer of Cloud Gate Dance Theater) and local residents, Chen established the

Hsin Kang Foundation of Culture and Education with the appeal of substituting the harmful cultures with something new. In 1988, Fengtian Temple in Hsin-Kang was chosen as the new destination for Mazu's[3] annual pilgrimage from Jennan Temple in Dajia, Taichung. This annual pilgrimage became the most important spiritual event in Hsin-Kang. During the pilgrimage, more than 100,000 followers from other parts of the country visited four major villages in Hsin-Kang, which naturally produced large amounts of trash from tourists and ash from fireworks. In consequence, the Foundation started to pay attention to the community's environment with the mobilization of volunteer workers cleaning the streets both during the pilgrimages and on a weekly basis.

Later, due to the air pollution from nearby factories in 1994 and the damage caused by Jiji Earthquake in Hsin-Kang in 1999, healthcare was added to the Foundation's concern. The Foundation has been collaborating with local residents to build a healthy shared space since then. In 2003, SARS haunted Taiwan. Chen recalls the "community turn" in Taiwan's new medical education after SARS: "Since then, medical specialists and community organizers collaboratively took the idea of 'community medicine' into actions. The 'community turn' was a deep criticism on the distanced medical specialist vision that views patients individualistically as if patients existed in isolation and detached their environments. Community medicine relies on a thorough care of a person, her family, and her community instead of just a diagnosis of one single physical illness. A person's illness is always already related to her mode of living, her family, and her community environment. Physical health and psychological health are two sides of the same coin." Chen adds that community medicine must be practiced on five levels of prevention based on the knowledge of preventive healthcare: (1) to promote and maintain the person's daily health, (2) to solidify the person's daily health with special protections, (3) to diagnose a disease and undergo a treatment early, (4) to prevent the person from having sequelae, and (5) to help the person return to her community after recovery. After this "community turn" in medical education, Chen has invited more than a thousand post-graduate year practitioners to visit Hsin-Kang to learn community medicine in practice.

In mid-February, people in Hsin-Kang were preparing for Mazu's pilgrimage scheduled in March when Covid-19 started to impact Taiwan. Chen persuaded the public to

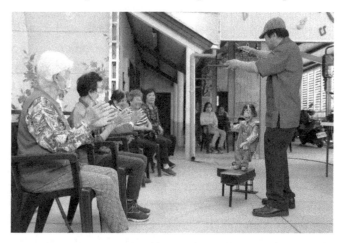

Figure 4.1   The Minnan marionette is performed to elders in Hsin-Kang. (Photo courtesy of the Hsin Kang Foundation of Culture and Education)

postpone the pilgrimage with an emphasis on the experience of cluster transmissions in Wanjia Feast (translation: Ten-Thousand-Families Feast)[4] in Wuhan and the South Korean church. With Chen's unremitting insistence and a wide public support, the postponement of Mazu's pilgrimage was finally announced on February 27. Afterwards, Covid-19 prevention in Hsin-Kang has continued to strengthen.

With a good number of single-elder, duo-elder and grandparent rearing families, a web of care around elders formed before Covid-19. The community-based Fuyuan Association established by Chin-Huang Chen has been forming this web of care since 2005. The volunteer workers in the Association deliver meals to the elders' homes every day and make routine phone calls to elders to keep up-to-date with their health conditions. They run blood pressure measuring stations once a week and health supply stations once a month at several locations in the community to provide elders with all of the facilities they need. These stations are also shared spaces for social gathering and exchanging knowledge about Covid-19. For the grandparent rearing families, grandchildren play a key role in elders' healthcare. Jingwen Wang, a volunteer at the Hsin Kang Foundation who was previously the Principle of Hsin-Kang Elementary School, choreographed an "anti-pandemic dance[5]" based on a Minnan-Taiwanese pop song. Wang taught the dance to children and asked them to teach their grandparents. The knowledge about Covid-19 prevention is communicated through the rhythmic body movements of the dancers.

Additionally, the volunteer workers of the Hsin Kang Foundation run a mobile library car at many locations in Hsin-Kang, especially those in remote areas, to share books with children and elders. Many picture books are useful for the illiterate elders. Sometimes, the mobile library car stops by a temple and provides Minnan marionette shows to reinvigorate the folk culture. A shared space for social gathering and exchanging knowledge about Covid-19 is created around the mobile library car. The mobile library car, books and volunteer workers have been routinely sanitized during the pandemic. The returning books all go through a sanitizing machine before they are put back onto bookshelves.

Chen says, "Elders are afraid of having no one to talk to. They are also afraid of being deemed as useless persons. The mutual supports among elders are therefore an indispensable part of our communal care. For one thing, elders find their value in helping others. For another, they listen to each other's voices." Chen invites elders to gather freely at Sohng[6] (translation: The Plain Garden), a shared space named after the nickname of Chen's mother, Ah-So.[7] Chen says, "We have a sister here in her 60s cooking for elders at Sohng. She has severe rheumatoid arthritis and is always in pain, but she still insists on cooking for others. 'When you take care of others, you forget your pain' – this is her attitude."

Besides elders, (im)migrants are another main concern in Hsin-Kang community. The (im)migrants from Southeast Asia and China suffer from racial stigmatization countrywide during this Covid-19 outbreak. Fuyuan Association and Hsin Kang Foundation are in collaboration with translators to assist (im)migrants in understanding Covid-19 preventive methods and fight against stigmatization. Chen highlights that many immigrant spouses who have become an organic part of the community volunteer themselves to help new immigrants settle into their new home.

Chen concludes, "While the government should be putting out fires, the civilians of local communities should eliminate the fire hazard. We've been making our community sustainable, and we'll continue our work."

J. Temple

Let's follow Mr. Hsieh, a temple manager and a spiritual healer, to take a look at the community in J. Temple, located on the outskirts of metropolitan Taipei.[8] Hsieh says, "Most visitors in J. Temple are long-term believers who have been connecting with spirituality for generations. A hiking trail nearby brings us random hikers as well. Thus, our community is majorly constituted by the long-term believers that are mutually acquainted and trusted, yet open to anyone who is interested." People in J. Temple started Covid-19 preventions a few weeks before the government's order. They reduced the entrances down to two people and designed an orderly foot traffic flow to ensure safe physical distance between individuals. A good number of medical masks had been stored in J. Temple before the Covid-19 outbreak due to the experience of SARS in 2003 and the air pollution in the city. In the midst of Covid-19, the managers in J. Temple have masks on, and they give a few masks away to each visitor for free.

The weekly gathering at their Sunday lunch buffet in the temple has unfortunately been suspended.

J. Temple is a shared space for pantheist Daoism. Hsieh introduces the caretakers: "In our temple, the Divine Doctor Huatuo[9] and the Divine Doctor Bianque[10] take care of those who have physical illnesses or insomnia. Jiutian Xuannu[11] and Samthaitsu[12] take care of those who have psychological trauma." As a spiritual healer, Hsieh sees himself as a translator between gods and people. He explains, "We follow Laozi's[13] Daoism. We believe that beings and things in the world interrelate with each other in a good balance. We call a state of good balance 'nature.'" I asked about the relation between human and nature, and he replies, "Human *is* nature. Everything is nature. Human and nature are not different entities. They have no different identities. Nature is not only the state of balance, but also the shared space for interrelated things and beings. Human beings cannot detach from nature." People in J. Temple believe that a person has to reflect on herself, refine herself, and find her own balance in nature when she is physically or psychologically ill. Hsieh says, "As a healer, what I do is assist a person find her balance." Hsieh points out that every pandemic is Wenshen's (translation: the God of Plague) practice of bringing a new balance in nature. A healer would help an ill person negotiate with Wenshen to give this person a chance to refine herself. "All is in a chain, you know. If a person does not behave in good conscience, she would be psychologically unbalanced; after that, her body would follow and become ill. She would move herself further and further away from nature. What a healer does is to break this negative chain, but the person has to create a positive chain after healing. That is how a rooted problem is solved. It would be useless to seek help from a healer if we do not do our job. We need to better ourselves. The gods will then help us, and nature will echo with us."

ALTERNATIVE IMAGINATIONS OF THE "FRONTLINE"

Usually, people imagine the medical practitioners in the emergency rooms and intensive care units to be on the "frontline" during the pandemic. With full respect for these practitioners, in this section, I invite you to think: are there other indispensable participants on the "frontline?" How do these participants form a web of communal support? How do we reshape our imagination of the "frontline" with full regard for these participants? When we call for public support for people on the "frontline" have we neglected some participants there?

The participants at the hospital entrance and the Covid-19 testing center

Let's follow En-Ju Kuo to take a look at the community at the hospital entrance of the Covid-19 testing center. Kuo works at the public affairs office in Asia University Hospital in Taichung. During the Covid-19 outbreak, most of the non-medical staff from each administrative office, like Kuo, take turns to run the Covid-19 testing center purposely located at the hospital entrance to limit virus transmission among patients and medical staff.

Around two to five practitioners are at the testing center during each shift, depending on how busy it is. Kuo highlights that *every* visitor coming to the hospital, no matter the purpose of the visit, has to be sanitized and tested for body temperature. Every visitor must also present her travel history recorded on her national health insurance card. The practitioners all wear masks, goggles, gloves and coveralls during the tests.

"The testing center was formed quickly in our hospital right after the Covid-19 outbreak in late January," Kuo explains, "immediately afterward was February, the key month for preventions. Our preventions in February enabled us to be relatively safe when Covid-19 went global. In February, my coworkers in the public affairs office and I did a lot of 'handicrafts.'" By "handicrafts," Kuo means the posted signs, arrows and numbers for smoothing foot traffic flow at the hospital entrance and in the hospital building, and posters that show updated policies and preventive methods.

Kuo says, "We are at the frontline, encounter visitors who might need our help. We have to be geared up at all times. Besides the practitioners at the testing center, the security officer at the hospital entrance also plays an essential part on this 'frontline.'" He checks if visitors have their masks on and directs them to the correct routes. He makes the testing process efficient and orderly. He also helps with the communications between visitors and practitioners. He wears full protection gear just like the practitioners. Kuo adds that the volunteer workers in the hospital, mostly the retired elders who want to support their neighborhood, are also pivotal on this "frontline."

Kuo believes that the meticulous collaboration among the practitioners in the testing center, the security officer, and the volunteers is an indispensable element for controlling the Covid-19 outbreak. Similar kinds of collaboration have been formed in other hospitals throughout Taiwan. "Out of fear of being infected, some people alienate, or even discriminate against whoever works at a hospital. I hope more people recognize the hard work in the hospital community and stop discrimination."

Kuo's other job is to receive and distribute donations from local communities. She conveys people's solidarity with the frontline. "People's inquiries and encouragements reach me through different mediums, such as phone calls, local legislators, health bureau, and fan-pages on the internet. I would confirm the delivery time and arrange proper distribution of donated supplies to the chief nurse officers in each unit. Usually the emergency rooms and intensive care units are prioritized." The supplies come in a great variety, including N95 masks, hand lotion and hand soap, various kinds of food and drink, and hand-made cards from children in the kindergarten nearby. Kuo notes, "Tea came in with warm and iced options. Women on their periods and elders can have warm ones. And we received two thousand pieces of dumpling in six flavors, including vegan. These details show people's warmest care."

Wheel pie makers

The wheel pie makers[14] at Mr. Wheel Restaurant in Taipei donated about 3,000 wheel pies to hospitals. The team

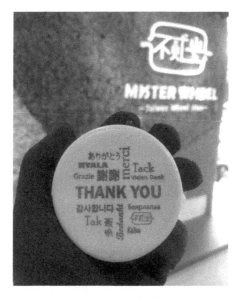

Figure 4.2 Taiwanese wheel pies stamped
with the "thank you" note were donated to
the hospitals in Taipei. (Photo courtesy of
Mr. Wheel Restaurant)

made about 200 wheel pies a day and stamped the "thank
you" note in 14 languages on the surface of those pies. Mr.
Li, the owner of Mr. Wheel Restaurant, says, "We asked
chief nurse officers to distribute our pies. We wish the ones
who have the heaviest workload would be prioritized, but
we never intervene in the process of distribution. Also,
we're not selective about which hospitals we deliver to. We
started with the ones closer to our restaurant, and then
expanded our delivery map. We did prioritize the ones
that have emergency rooms, though. Pies were delivered
equally to small and big hospitals. It's noteworthy that
the big hospitals generally do not need donations, while

the small ones do. We should show stronger solidarity to small hospitals." Li adds that his team once sent 100 wheel pies to a press conference held by the Taiwan Centers for Disease Control, and 50 of those pies were specifically for journalists and reporters. "We're thankful to them. They're also on the frontline."

Field reporters and journalists

Field reporters and journalists are essential workers during the outbreak. They are on the frontline passing on timely information, speeding ahead to compete with the rapidly growing pandemic. Mr. Yu, a cameraman, visited a hospital in Taipei to cover preparation of isolation rooms with negative air pressure a few weeks after the outbreak in Wuhan. He followed the hospital policy to wear coveralls, an N95 mask, goggles and gloves. He is concerned about the stigmatization of reporters and journalists due to the commercialization of journalism, polarized party politics, and growing patriotism after the legacy of the Cold War. Reporters and journalists – *jizhe*[15] in Mandarin – are often vilified as prostitutes – also *jizhe*[16] in Mandarin – with a word play of different Chinese written characters that share the same pronunciation. In the midst of Covid-19, this stigmatization got wilder. Several reporters and journalists who asked the state governors harsh or investigative questions have been doxed and bullied on the internet. Yu recalls, "My peer even got punched when he was taking photos of people in a queue receiving masks distributed by the government ... I mean, of course journalists and reporters should do better. When the whole journalism industry is unbearably commercialized, we share the responsibility to resist. But I wish people, including my family and friends, would stand in solidarity with us when we resist. At least, I hope they try to understand our difficulties. If the whole industry and the audience's attitudes do not change, our resistance would be in vain. Getting punched and doxed have been happening before the pandemic. This pandemic just makes us more aware of the unfriendly attitudes addressed toward us."

CODA: ENVISIONING SPACES BEYOND STATE BORDERS

This is a conclusive note on problematizing the state borders during a pandemic. While the numbers of deaths and confirmed Covid-19 cases in Taiwan are relatively low in the global scale, the discriminative discourse is not mild. The racist scapegoating of Chinese and Southeast Asians during this pandemic epitomizes the revival of the Cold War structure in new forms of imperiality and coloniality. Some collective voices in Taiwan call for an understanding of people beyond state borders.

Saving lives equally and making unharmful relationalities

In mid-March, 13 scholars from Academia Sinica and different universities in Taiwan petitioned the public to stop discrimination in their public statement titled "Saving Lives Equally and Making Unharmful Relationalities."[17] They call for a radical change of the ongoing discrimination towards people who travel or migrate across the state borders between Taiwan and China. Diverse supporters in and outside of Taiwan signed this petition. Nonetheless, the petition statement was harshly criticized and debated.

Here is a summary of the five appeals in the petition statement: (1) Stop justifying discrimination in the name of pandemic prevention. Stop calling Covid-19 discriminative names that reproduce the racial discrimination towards Chinese and Asians in Western societies. If the virus is universally contagious regardless of a person's nationality, ethnicity, sex and sexual orientation, healthcare should be universally provided as well. (2) We should perceive people and the state separately and support people across the state borders. (3) While we see the Chinese state as a bully, we don't need to dismiss every single thing about Chinese people. (4) People as well as the state in Taiwan should take the feelings of the peoples in China, Hong Kong and Macao into consideration when they take any actions. The cultural affinity and geographical neighboring among us should not be ignored. (5) We should revive kindness and politeness in ourselves and get rid of our violent language.

Chih-Ming Wang, an associate researcher in Academia Sinica, who co-wrote the petition statement, describes the lack of mutual understanding between the Taiwanese and Chinese as the head-on crash of two trains dashing into the globalized contemporary realm from two opposite sides of the Cold War structure. On the one side, the Chinese have experienced a post-socialist turn of their state since the 1980s. Their colonial memories were incorporated into the state-oriented nationalist discourse of "one hundred years of humiliation,"[18] which serves as justification for the state's imperial turn. On the other side, the nationalist postcolonial discourse has been rapidly growing in Taiwan. Various sorts of anti-colonial imaginations (e.g. Third World solidarity) have been marginalized under the dominant nationalist discourse. All in all, the dominant discourses on both sides, in Wang's view, are over-simplifying the complexity of coloniality and erasing the anti-colonial imaginations that are not favored by any states. Wang concludes, "The imagined community in the dominant discourse today might not be able to help us build a people-centered imagined community in reality. The questions about borders are hard to answer, but is it really necessary to think about people with the presumption of borders? We need other imaginations."

NOTES

1. Original text: 大家樂
2. Original text: 電子花車
3. Original text: 媽祖
4. Original text: 萬家宴
5. The title of the dance is "Hsin Kang IN, virus OUT."
6. Original text: 素園
7. Original text: 阿素
8. Hsieh depicts the surroundings of J. Temple with his poem: "Sitting leisurely in the temple's yard, I am surrounded by sweetly fragrant osmanthus. I gaze afar at Yangming Mountain, the blue sky, and the green water of Waishuang River. When the rain rests and a neon sky ladder appears, I realize the balance in nature that cannot be expressed in words." Original text: 暇坐倚廟埕木樨,　觀遠山天藍綠溪；雨歇跨霓虹天梯,　且忘聞大道歸悉
9. Original text: 華陀神醫
10. Original text: 扁鵲神醫

11. Original text: 九天玄女
12. Original text: 三太子
13. Original text: 老子
14. Original text: 車輪餅
15. Original text: 記者
16. Original text: 妓者
17. Original text: 救無別類，應物無傷
18. Original term: 百年國恥

CHAPTER FIVE

Standing in Solidarity with Those Who Must Refuse to Keep Social Distance: Disability Activism in South Korea

Ji Young Shin (translated by Han Gil Jang)

THE MARCH OF THE SEGREGATED

> Say no to social distancing. Although we'd have to keep physical distance, we must socially stick together and stand in solidarity! (Pak Kyŏngsŏk)

> We have gathered here again today, as if we had never been discriminated against, as if we had never lost hope ... We felt so much pain as we saw on the news the patients dying behind the closed doors of psychiatric wards ... We are all standing here today because we fought our way out, and were able to come out the other end. (Chang Hyeyŏng)

Strict social distancing rules were still in place in South Korea on April 20 when a group of disability activists and people with disabilities flooded onto the streets of Seoul, marched and rallied under the slogan "Physical

Distancing for Covid-19, Social Solidarity for CHORUS-20," maintaining a 2-meter distance from each other. Ten days have passed since that day, and with May Day fast approaching, a sense of relief is in the air, as the number of newly confirmed cases of Covid-19 has gone down to zero – a major accomplishment achieved in 72 days since the outbreak in which over 6,000 people became infected within two weeks in the city of Daegu. The officials have credited strict implementation of social distancing and everyday preventive measures for this accomplishment.[1]

Internationally, South Korea has been praised for bringing Covid-19 under control, and the secrets to such success have been identified as making widely available the Covid-19 testing kits, implementing strict social distancing rules and ensuring transparency with the public. In fact, such measures did seem to have prevented hoarding or medical system breakdown, and therefore provided an ideal case for observing what kind of changes in the forms of social relations Covid-19 prevention and control brought about.

The most noteworthy observation concerns the flip side of social distancing: strict implementation of social distancing rules exacerbated the conditions of those who had already been segregated. The homeless, the poor and contract workers – especially women – became deprived of the means of survival, while immigrant workers and refugees were forced to head home or move to another country in spite of the risk of imminent persecution. The new moral imperative of social distancing brought about enforced solitude on the tacit consensus that it was inevitable. In a way, the entire society became subject to "cohort isolation."

Most of the major Covid-19 outbreaks occurred in certain religious communities, secure wards for people with disabilities and nursing homes. On February 23, when the confirmed cases of Covid-19 rose to 566, 111 of them were held in the psychiatric ward in Cheongdo Daenam Hospital. A striking fact was that even though 98 percent of the patients in the closed psychiatric ward were diagnosed with Covid-19, none of their family members or relatives were infected. The quarantine lasted for over a month, during which time the patients were in effect prisoned in the ward that wasn't even partitioned. Thus, the virus was "contained within the borders of the closed ward."[2]

The first death from Covid-19 in South Korea was a man hospitalized for over 20 years in a psychiatric ward in Daenam Hospital. At the time of his death, his body weighed only 42 kilograms, which, along with his symptoms, made it clear that the awful living conditions almost certainly contributed to his death as much as the virus. His body was cremated swiftly without autopsy, which Pak Kyŏngsŏk, from the National Council of Popular School for People with Disability, criticized as treating people with disabilities as carriers of the virus and segregating and subjecting them to cohort isolation in the name of welfare.[3] After a series of protests, the patients in the closed psychiatric wards in Daenam Hospital were relocated to other hospitals. In other words, they became deinstitutionalized only insofar as they were infected or dead.

The presence of those who couldn't afford to keep social distance has laid bare the forms of segregation and exclusion that have been in place long before the outbreak of Covid-19. The sense of frustration that non-disabled people have felt during lockdown has been prescribed to people with disabilities as their condition of life.[4] As many of them are unable to carry out their daily affairs without caregivers, the imperative of social distancing implies not only another form of institutionalization that they fought so hard to reject, but also something close to a death sentence.

Therefore, the April 20 rally was also a moment in which the solidarity among "different bodies" revealed how the very fear of Covid-19 was the normative, as it was rooted in racism and eugenics that excluded the bodies that deviated from the socially normative view. The march was slow, and oftentimes the participants let out indistinguishable cries into the air. The stage at the rally was filled with dancing bodies. The dancing, staggering bodies at the CHORUS-20 posed a major challenge to the normative view on disability and illness.[5]

For people with disabilities who have long been socially segregated, there is no "normal life" to go back to. Thus, the movement for solidarity during the era of pandemic began by refusing to keep social distance, and necessitates envisioning post-Covid-19 from the non-normative perspective on disability and illness.

To learn from those who couldn't afford to keep social distance, I met with disability activists in Daegu, known as the epicenter of the Covid-19 outbreak in South Korea. The following is a record of those who stood in solidarity with one another as they fought the threat of double institutionalization brought about by the pandemic.

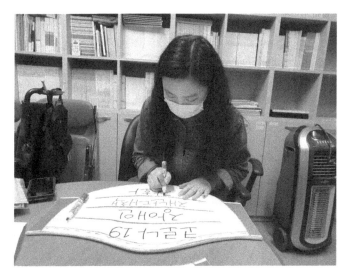

Figure 5.1　Kwon Suchin working on a placard that reads: "Proper COVID-19 Relief for People with Disabilities!" (Photo courtesy of the author)

FROM SOCIAL DISTANCE TO SOCIAL BONDS

Cho Minche, administrative director at Changaein jiyŏkkongdongch'e (Local Community for People with Disabilities) in Daegu, is in charge of reaching out to and cooperating with governmental and civil society organizations and activist groups in providing support for people with disabilities who are subject to self-isolation or diagnosed with Covid-19. Cho claimed that public welfare often fails to account for many of the people with disabilities, many of whom therefore are not reflected in the official statistics.

On February 20, it was announced that around 20 people, 13 with disabilities, had been in close contact with a confirmed case of Covid-19 at Taegusaram changaein charipsaenghwalsentŏ (Daegu Center for Disability Independent Living). Another individual with developmental disability at Tarittol charipsaenghwalsentŏ (Tarittol Center for Independent Living) was diagnosed with Covid-19 on February 20, which put his housemate in self-isolation. Even though many of the people with disabilities in Daegu weren't able to practice self-isolation, the city of Daegu never implemented any measures in this regard. As the caregivers became increasingly subject to self-isolation, people began to avoid working as caregivers out of fear. As the welfare institutions stopped adherence to social distancing rules, the infrastructure for supporting people with disabilities came to a halt. Cho recalled that until the implementation of emergency caregiving services, no public support was available for two weeks as the entire social welfare infrastructure was situated in the private sector.[6]

Caregiving support ceased, which official statistics failed to reflect, as people with disabilities still carried on. In the end, activists began to isolate together with people with disabilities who were diagnosed with Covid-19, and other activists who weren't subject to self-isolation kept reaching out to the public sector and civil society to create plans and protocols.

Over twelve hours, from 5 am to 5 pm, the activists at our organization provided care while people were making calls to the city and the Ministry of Health and Welfare to secure hospital beds. Also, you know, people with developmental disabilities will need assistance and communication aids, and what was disappointing was that they had nothing prepared in that regard, so we had to come up with and provide a protocol book for that.[7]

Cho assessed that it was their strong collective bonds that helped them overcome such challenges. Social distancing is a type of preventive measure that operates by severing the ties between bodies. However, Cho's experience illuminates the fact that the pandemic prevention measures must involve forming strong social bonds instead of social distancing. In fact, Cho was familiar with this lesson as he engaged with disability studies scholars in Japan in 2011 and learned about the predicaments that the people with disabilities face during times of disaster. Even before there were any confirmed cases in South Korea, Cho's organization, along with four others, convened, prepared supplies such as masks, rehearsed disaster management measures, and made necessary requests to the local government. Although there weren't enough hospital beds to accommodate them in Daegu, the activists got in contact with the Solidarity Against Disability Discrimination's Seoul branch and successfully secured hospital beds for the five people in Seoul and Gyeongbuk province. Help also came from the disability community, as people learned about the circumstances in Daegu via social networks and began sending medical supplies and non-perishable foods worth approximately $123,000. The total amount of donations from all over the country, including the one from eBay Korea, added up to over $110,000.[8]

During this period, Cho has received many phone calls regarding donations as the disability organizations became a hub of medical supplies and disaster support. He particularly recalled the children who sent handwritten letters of support and the artists who donated their exhibition revenue. Cho confessed an ambivalence to all the support during a disaster, noting the past complaints they received during disability rights rallies.

It is striking the amount of support and solidarity disability activists were able to garner in Daegu. Cho emphasized that the conservative political atmosphere in Daegu might have driven them to strive harder for deinstitutionalization and implementation of caregiving support, as well as to form stronger bonds. Kwŏn Suchin at the Tarittol Support Center also claimed that the disability activists have formed a close relationship with not only the anti-poverty activists but also immigrant women and workers, and children's rights activists.[9] Standing in solidarity with one another during the times of Covid-19 would have been difficult without their experience and the network they have worked so hard to establish.

At the same time, there were risks associated with working closely during the Covid-19 outbreak, some of which manifested in a way that accentuated the difference between non-disabled activists and activists with disabilities. Many activists with disabilities in Daegu, it turned out, began to show symptoms of depression:

The activist leaders who have disabilities were encouraged to stay home because, you know, the situation is extremely grim for those with disabilities who are diagnosed with Covid-19. They later told us about how they felt so powerless as a leader and a member of the organization, in addition to the sense of fear in the times of pandemic.[10]

This begs the question of what the aims of ongoing movements for solidarity must be. Stopping at an "aid package" and "welfare" implies a return to the "state of constant disaster" for those with disabilities, which has been in place long before Covid-19. Instead, the disability activists call for "more than mere survival" and strengthening social bonds, especially, during times of pandemic.

REJECTING THE REINSTITUTIONALIZATION OF THE DEINSTITUTIONALIZED

Chŏng Chiwŏn works for Tarittol, where he has been helping Mr. KC (pseudonym) with independent living, until KC was diagnosed with Covid-19 and hospitalized. When KC's housemate, Mr. KT (pseudonym), was subject to self-isolation, Chŏng joined him to provide assistance. Kwŏn, in charge of overseeing Tarittol's residential facilities for independent living, has been an activist for ten years.

While the rest of the society were trying their best to stay away from those diagnosed with Covid-19, Chŏng and Kwŏn chose to stay with those who were diagnosed or in close proximity with them. Their choice reveals that those who can't afford to keep social distance are in need of companionship, rather than stopping short at providing material support. An acute awareness of their pace of life and their words is essential, which also sheds light on preventing not only reinstitutionalization of the deinstitutionalized but also institutionalizing the entire society.

While Chŏng subjected himself to self-isolation with Mr. KT, he constantly provided support for him while cleaning the space three times a day and airing it out every two hours. When asked whether he felt worried about himself, he answered that the only thing he had in mind was wishing him well.

> Mr. KT has been institutionalized for several decades, and I think the self-isolation period, although it only lasted two weeks, reminded him of those years ... I think he felt frustrated as to why he should be doing all this, in spite of the coronavirus and all, so I kept explaining to him over and over again and provided support – especially mental support ... When he gets mad or worried, I told him over and over that everything was okay, encouraging him.[11]

In Chŏng's experience, we get a glimpse of what deinstitutionalized self-isolation might look like. The part where Chŏng explained things to KT "over and over" is especially suggestive. As Chŏng groped for words that were more intelligible to KT, KT became willing to accept and overcome his situation, even if not fully understanding the impact of Covid-19.

Kwŏn's words also provide insights into the strategies of social bonding and companionship during the times of pandemic. Kwŏn described how the activists at Tarittol have been doing the rounds of disinfection at five of Tarittol's residential houses for independent living from 9 am to 6 pm, seven days a week.

> I felt sorry for the activists who are working full-time, and I also worried about not providing adequate support for Mr. KC ... Even so, in the end, when I look back ... I realized that no one but we could have done it ... We were working all night to come up with ways to provide support for Mr. KC, but there was no help from the city or the district office.[12]

Clearly, Kwŏn has faith in her coworkers. At the same time, Kwŏn expressed feelings of guilt over how this has affected her fellow workers with disabilities. At one point, she suggested to one of her coworkers who had motor disability to work from home, as she believed that people with motor disabilities were more vulnerable to Covid-19. After working from home for two weeks, he came back to work looking depressed and discouraged. While telecommuting, he could not help but compare himself negatively to the non-disabled activists who often engaged in physical labor.

> None of us were so well prepared for this, and we were too busy dealing with the situation that we weren't able to care for each other and consider how we felt as much as we wanted to ... Just like that. It makes me keep

crying like this ... I guess this isn't just my problem. We probably need to see a psychiatrist. All of us working here full-time ... [13]

Standing in solidarity with one another also involves taking a closer look at relationships that have been formed, which are full of pain, joy, frustration and empathy. In this light, Kwŏn's experience during the pandemic culminates in the realization of how the pandemic affects the movement for independent living. While strict social distancing rules were in place, activists had to maintain even closer contact with the residents at their facilities, which served as an opportunity for a closer look at their lives and the reality of living with disabilities. In one instance, Kwŏn went to provide support for someone with developmental disability at the residential house, prepared all three meals and left for the day. When she came back that night, she found her care receiver hadn't – and couldn't – eat. Oftentimes, people with developmental disabilities who have spent a long time at institution need to be reminded to eat meals and take medicine.

Disability policymaking in South Korea takes into account only the physical capabilities of care receivers, which is part of the reason why caregiving support is provided only for three to four hours a day for people with developmental disabilities. Kwŏn's account captures the moment in which the activists became, again, reminded of the fact that the current state of policymaking renders independent living extremely difficult. Such a "discovery" is, ironically, made possible because of the Covid-19 outbreak. Kwŏn spoke as she tried to hold back her tears:

"This ... I know we're working to change policies and all, but (sobs) ... things don't change so easily, and the work here ... (keeps sobbing) isn't easy."[14]

The interview with Kwŏn also suggests the need to be cautious of the tendencies that reinforce institutionalization, which became widespread as the pandemic intensified. Chŏng shared a story of a person with disabilities who, living in a high-rise apartment, was subject to self-isolation. When other residents at the apartment became aware that there was a person with disabilities who was subject to self-isolation, they demanded to know

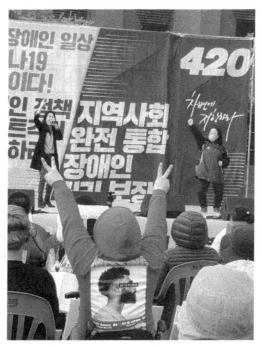

Figure 5.2 People dancing on stage with singer Im Chŏngtŭk. (Photo courtesy of the author)

his identity, requested disinfection of the entire building, and expressed outright bigotry. This story indicates that the tendencies that reinforce institutionalization arise from the exclusion of people with disabilities in the local community: while people send help and sympathize with people with disabilities with whom they are not directly involved, they also seek to exclude and express hatred towards their neighbors who have disabilities and are subject to self-isolation. The story also begs the question of how solidarity can help dismantle these tendencies.

APPROPRIATION OF COHORT ISOLATION INTO SOCIAL BONDING

As a vast number of people in the city of Daegu were subject to self-isolation, the Ministry of Health and Welfare announced that people with disabilities who are subject to self-isolation will be provided with 24-hour caregiving or placed in quarantine facilities.[15] However, only the homeless and non-citizens were placed in the quarantine facilities in the end, and the 24-hour caregiving service was hardly available.[16] Under such circumstances, Kim Sihyŏng, an activist at Taegusaram changaein charipsaenghwalsentŏ who has brain lesions, decided to go into self-isolation alone. He recalled, "Well, my conditions aren't so severe (laughs) ... So I decided to do it on my own."[17]

During the self-isolation period, he received a phone call every day at 10 am from the district office and reported his body temperature. He was also in charge of reporting on the statuses of other people with disabilities who were subject to self-isolation in the vicinity. It took him two hours to shower, usually 20 minutes with a caregiver. Kim had to crawl to the door to get the food that was left. What angered him, however, was the bag of groceries that the district office has sent, which contained raw rice and cabbages – foods that Kim could not cook on his own.

Many reporters requested interviews with Kim as they wanted to feature a story of a person with a disability who was subject to self-isolation. Some of them lacked even the most basic understanding of what it means to live with disabilities, and others attempted staging for dramatic effects. Kim was determined to use every opportunity to inform the public of the reality of a person with disabilities subject to self-isolation. He added that had he become diagnosed with Covid-19, he would have had more stories to share with the public.

As the first three deaths from Covid-19 in South Korea were all people with disabilities, Kim was extremely worried as he went into self-isolation. However, he still claimed that getting infected with Covid-19 couldn't be worse than being isolated and unable to receive support as a person with disability. His remarks were hopeful:

At least, there still are cases where people recover from the coronavirus … During the MERS outbreak, or even the influenza pandemic, not that many people with disabilities were affected, because they were all institutionalized or stuck at home … the reason why people with disabilities get infected is because they come into contact with others … The people with disabilities actually live in the local communities, and that's why they catch the disease, and that's why the government acknowledges us … In the past, the epidemic has swerved and bypassed us in the big institutions, but now, in the big cities, they get infected.[18]

BODIES THAT REFUSE INSTITUTIONALIZATION

In spite of its accomplishments, the imposition of social distancing reinforced institutionalizationist tendencies. As a result, those with disability and/or illness – for whom social distancing proved to be life-threatening – were silenced in the name of pandemic control, which was oriented towards the so-called healthy and normal body. Meanwhile, disability activists have refused to comply with social distancing and strove to reach out. Their activities shed light on what it means to stand in solidarity in times of pandemic.

One of the important insights from their activities is what the "non-normative" body is capable of. Kwŏn confessed that she was surprised to see the people with developmental disabilities adapt so quickly to the changes brought by the pandemic. When KC was diagnosed with Covid-19, he seemed rather happy about being able to go outside.

In this light, what must be closely examined is Kim Sihyŏng's remark on the "swerving" of previous epidemics that "bypassed" him, affirming the possibility of solidarity among bodies with disabilities and illness. Konggam, an activist group for women with disabilities, described such bodies as "eccentric," which is also illuminated upon in a writing of one woman with disability who described how she has been striving for independent living:

I want to live a life where my disability isn't someone else's burden. I don't want to be reduced to a mere receiver of caregiving service. I want to be a person, breathing outside the borders of institutionalization … I always tell myself, that I shouldn't be afraid of being deflected off as my body with disability constantly seeks to be in motion and deinstitutionalized.[19]

Perhaps her writing teaches us how to stand in solidarity with "eccentric bodies" that are not afraid of being deflected off the institutionalizationist tendencies, which have been proliferating in times of pandemic. Currently, the South Korean society is transitioning from implementing social distancing to encouraging "everyday prevention measures." What is missing from this transition is the need to stand in solidarity with the eccentric bodies that are capable of forming new social bonds and to remain cautious of tendencies that avoid, exclude and segregate them. Perhaps the vaccine for such bigotry is in dire need at the moment, as it has been prior to the pandemic, and the key to that vaccine may be found in the solidarity with "eccentric bodies" that are not afraid of being deflected off the institutionalizational tendencies.

NOTES

1. Yi Hyein, "K'orona19 chiyŏksahoe hwakchin 31pŏn hwak-chinja ihu 72il man" [COVID-19 and Local Communities: 72 Days After the 31st Confirmed Case], *Kyŏnghyang sinmun*, April 30, 2020, http://news.khan.co.kr/kh_news/khan_art_view.html?artid=202004301658001&code=

940100#csidx9b27afc8a88a4a99b13a7408476bfb0 (accessed May 2, 2020).

2. Yu Kihun, "P'yeswaebyŏngdong k'orona19, chiptan kamnyŏm kamch'uŏjin chilmundŭl" [COVID-19 in Closed Ward: Hidden Truth Behind COVID-19 Outbreak], *beminor*,February23,2020,https://beminor.com/detail.php?number=14398&thread=04r04 (accessed May 2, 2020).

3. Pak Sŭngwŏn, "Changaein'gŏjushisŏl k'ohot'ŭ kyŏngninŭn chiptan'gamyŏm k'iunŭn kkol' in'gwŏnwi chinjŏng" [Appeal to Human Rights Committee: "Cohort Isolation of People with Disabilities Will Lead to Mass Infection"], *beminor*, February 26, 2020, https://beminor.com/detail.php?number=14398&thread=04r04 (accessed May 2, 2020).

4. Ko Pyŏngkwŏn, "Chaep'anijŏne naeryŏjin p'an'gyŏl" [Judgment Before Trial], in *Mungmuk*. 2018. Seoul: Tolbegae, 211.

5. The video documentation of the rally is available on: www.youtube.com/watch?v=Qb5eh5E3Kjs (accessed May 2, 2020).

6. Cho Minche in interview with the author, April 16, 2020.

7. Ibid.

8. Ibid.

9. Kwŏn Suchin in interview with the author, April 17, 2020.

10. Ibid.

11. Chŏng Chiwŏn in interview with the author, April 17, 2020.

12. Kwŏn.

13. Ibid.

14. Ibid.

15. Yi Pora, "Tandong: Pokchibu 'Changaein k'orona19 cha-gagyŏngnidoemyŏn 24shigan tolbomjiwŏn'" [Exclusive: Ministry of Health and Welfare Promises "24-Caregiving Service for People with Disabilities Diagnosed with COVID-19"], *Kyŏnghyang sinmun*, February 21, 2020, https://news.khan.co.kr/kh_news/khan_art_view.html?art_id=202002211715001&code=940601 (accessed May 2, 2020).

16. Yi Pora, "Taegu t'alshisŏl changaein k'orona19 hwakchin 'Chiwŏnillyŏng ŏpko kyŏngnishisŏl motka'" [When People with Disabilities on Independent Living in Daegu are Confirmed with COVID-19: "No Support, No Quarantine"], *Kyŏnghyang sinmun*, February 29, 2020, http://news.khan.co.kr/kh_news/khan_art_view.html?artid=202002291440001&code=940100#csidx0bf7319007a26 8bb00b812e026d6bce (accessed May 2, 2020).

17. Kim Sihyŏng in interview with the author, April 17, 2020.

18. Ibid.

19. Kim Sanghŭi, "Hwaltongbojo-Nanŭn namŭi soni p'iryohamnida" [Caregiving Assistance: I Need Someone Else's Hand], in Ŏtchŏmyŏn *isanghan mom* [Perhaps an Eccentric Body], ed. Changaeyŏsŏnggonggam. 2019. Paju, South Korea: Owŏrŭibom, 143.

CHAPTER SIX

Rethinking Minority and Mainstream in India

Debarati Roy

The Covid-19 pandemic has not only jeopardized people's health, but the lockdown worldwide is sparking key questions about the impact of pandemics and associated countermeasures on the global economy. India's economic damage is mounting, and the extension of the nationwide lockdown is drawing attention to the country's deep economic divide. Although the lockdown will affect everyone, it has already disproportionately hit the lives of the poor. The government states it is raising funds, but there are countless professionals and daily wage-earners in the country such as rickshaw pullers, tea stall owners, bus drivers, street vendors and construction workers who live as they earn daily. With the entire public transport system shutting down and a strict restriction on venturing out in public places, daily wage-earners have no means to earn. Moreover, images and videos of police officers forcing people to do squats, sit-ups and push-ups as public punishment, and in some situations, violently beating those who ignore the restrictions have been circulating on social media.

After Prime Minister Narendra Modi declared a ban on going outside in an attempt to contain the spread of Covid-19, millions of people are starting measures and solutions to address hunger, destitution and indefinite uncertainty. The country has a large floating population of migrant workers who have moved from villages to cities and across states for work. The news of this nationwide lockdown has put their lives into disarray, as industrial units and public places deemed non-essential have shut. Several images of migrants walking hundreds of kilometers to reach their homes across state borders have starkly emphasized the implications of a country in shutdown and its workforce in the unorganized economy.

Coupled with the issue of class divide, another offshoot of the Covid-19 conversation is the rise of Islamophobia. Several media sources have reported how the Covid-19 crisis has sparked online hate speeches and notes targeted at Muslims because of a few fake stories that are circulating on social media sites. Besides the overt or subtle messaging linking the pandemic to Islam, the measures taken by police including the tendency to suppress protests and civil society activism in the foreseeable future are also labeled to portray the government's authoritarian instincts.

Nonetheless, as India grapples with containing the coronavirus pandemic, stories of hope and solidarity are emerging from the country. The situation has underlined a crucial element – the power of solidarity, hope and humanity. What is particularly remarkable in this moment is how people from all sections of society have come together and organized mutual aid projects across the country.

In this chapter, I aim to give voice to and document the general public's efforts in building solidarity groups. While browsing through social media platforms, I came across a plethora of these inspiring initiatives. Then there were stories of people that did not find much prominence on social media. For instance, it was endearing to learn about how social status based on gender orientation could not restrict a marginal community from responding to the call for humanity. Several studies including ethnographic accounts show that the Hijra[1] community faces harsh discrimination; hijras (eunuch/transvestite) are an institutionalized third gender role in India. Hijra are neither male nor female but contain elements of both and are not only excluded from the mainstream society, they are often confined to an inhuman state. Historian Urvashi Butalia[2] notes that deprived of their traditional roles as caretakers of harems, their main occupations are the offering of blessings in return for money or begging or sex work. Most of them cannot seek employment anywhere, nor do many of them have the necessary documentation that marks them as citizens with entitlements and rights. Nonetheless, as Ayantika's narrative highlights, after the announcement of the lockdown, many hijras have come forward and initiated solidarity movements in their local areas. Similarly, Asif Ahmed's project undermines the Islamophobia controversy that is receiving ample screen space and time on several news channels across the country. In our conversation, he never brought up the issue of religion or hinted at how despite being a Muslim he is serving people across other religious faiths. Rather, he is committed to reach out to more neighborhoods despite knowing full well that his own business will take several months to regain momentum. In this chapter, I will highlight similar incredible community networks that aim to protect neighbors as well as strangers during the coronavirus pandemic.

HIJRA: CRISIS CHANGES PERCEPTIONS AND RELATIONSHIPS

One of my first interactions for this project was with an undergraduate student, Ayantika Maity. Ayantika is an inhabitant of Kolkata, West Bengal, and she is a third-year college student majoring in Statistics. I wanted to have a conversation with her to have a sense of what is going on in the city in terms of academics, professional work, mutual aid projects, and everyone transitioning and settling into a new routine. While the chunk of our conversation focused on solidarity initiatives, we also discussed the process of transitioning to online classes and how we might think of enhancing and cultivating our creative desires and capabilities now. Ayantika invites us to think of the important role that oppressed minorities are making, despite and maybe even because of their status.

ON LOCKDOWN AND ESSENTIALS

Ayantika begins by emphasizing that everything except essential services had closed. Daily grocery items are available. "Fresh food markets are open 6 am to 9 am. Big department stores like Big Bazaar and Spencer's have opted for the afternoon slot. While generally these hypermarkets would sell their items in bulk, now they have issued a limited amount. Some of these retail chains are offering grocery delivery service as well but the minimum purchase amount varies across stores. And in the open fresh food markets, the pricing has no logic."

ON STUDENTS TAKING INITIATIVE

Ayantika notes that the state government has issued an order for distributing rice and potatoes in different schools that provide mid-day meals[3] to students during regular academic session. So, these schools will supply food materials to students who are eligible for mid-day meals but are staying home due to the lockdown in the wake of coronavirus. Besides school administration committees, students are forming independent groups to initiate solidarity projects. Specifically, she talks about two of her former classmates who have shared a post on Facebook inviting people to contribute money via Google Pay. They intend to get essentials for people who are not able to manage a one-time meal. While initially not too many people expressed confidence, gradually, her classmates have received support from friends, neighbors and peers to continue with this work.

ON THE TRANSGENDER COMMUNITY COMING FORWARD

Ayantika says that hijras (recognized as a third gender in India) "had reached out to their community circles to raise money, and they came to local clubs to give food essentials including rice, lentils, and potatoes using this money."

Now, the club members are redistributing the food among the needy.

Ayantika draws attention to how a significant population of Indian society stigmatizes hijras. She says that we generally encounter hijras in public settings – such as when we see them boisterously dancing and singing while asking for money on a train or blessing a wedding. Ayantika shares how the very sight of a hijra would cause discomfort and fear in many people – there are people who say they extort money from parents of newborns, showing up at wedding functions and asking for money; they also have the reputation of harassing passengers on trains. They are believed to have the power to bestow or deny good fortune and fertility. As they approach people to ask for money, hijras typically clap in a distinct way with flat palms striking together at a perpendicular angle, and not in the usual way one usually applauds. Many say these claps are a form of protest against a society that does not recognize their existence.

Ayantika emphasizes that while distributing the food, club members said that a few hijras came to their club with essentials and told them that since they always ask for money when they visit households to shower blessings on newlyweds or babies, they wanted to give back to society. So, they donated money to help needy households.

EVERY INDIVIDUAL CAN HELP

Another student who was gracious to share his initiative is Dipayan Mazumder. In his final year of a master's program he works with the retail section of a popular Indian department store. I am a member of a public foodie group on Facebook, and one day as I was browsing through the feed, I came across his post:

> In this critical period, instead of using lots of costly ingredients to prepare extra-ordinary dishes and demonstrating our culinary skills, can't we just have simple food for every day and save the extra money for the weak? Let's make some regular items like rice, lentils, and chicken curry or anything that can make them full for the day (just one day a week by our family). Some people just need basic food to survive in this pandemic situation. Let's come forward and contribute one day to feed them. Post it here. Tag me and your friends. Feed beggars in your locality. (No politician or police will stop you to feed them).

I spoke with Dipayan about his background and what he and others are doing now to help those in need.

After the government announced strict lockdown, images of people's cooking adventures have flooded the internet. His girlfriend suggested that he might think of a public platform like this foodie group to post this note. Dipayan says that we often come across images of people's experiences with restaurant food or cooking something extraordinary at home. So why not encourage these people to come forward and take some steps to help?

Dipayan says that even before the Covid-19 scenario, as a child he always wanted to reach out to people to offer help in terms of food and money. He specifies that he is not involved with any organization. Rather, he collaborates with his girlfriend and a few other friends. He remembers that on their anniversary his girlfriend proposed not having a grand anniversary celebration. "So, instead of going to hotels and restaurants, she suggested that we could offer food to people who would be in need. I readily agreed, and we went ahead with this thought; our friends, too, became part of this." They did something similar when one of his friends was getting married; noticing leftover food, they redistributed it to those in need. He reiterates that instead of spending money on bars and restaurants, we can make the simplest food and distribute amongst the needy.

ON COVID-19 ENDEAVOR

Dipayan had some savings and he and his girlfriend began. Her mother cooked food for a huge number of people, and Dipayan took the initiative to distribute the food. However, not too many people are staying on the streets so he rode around the neighborhood to see if people were in need.

SIMILAR INITIATIVES IN THE NEIGHBORHOOD

Elderly people in his residential complex have organized together to collect money so they can purchase and distribute food items. "They are not cooking food but trying to buy rice and potatoes. Then they are wrapping these items in bags and giving to people. But the issue is that they are not going to the slums or outside of their neighborhood. They are standing outside of the residential building because the police will stop them if they walk around in the streets. So, somehow, they are not able to help them who actually need it."

He has also noticed that in some areas people are not able to avail themselves of cooking gas because of delivery issues. So, delivering cooked food becomes essential.

Besides this, a few women in his neighborhood are making masks in bulk using stitching machines. "They are selling these masks to the party office for INR 5, and the latter is giving these masks to the common people for free. First, masks are not readily available and the ones that the local medical shops are selling could be expensive. So, this is really helpful for a lot of people. Also, it gives these women an opportunity to get involved in good work and also make some earnings; however little the earning could be, it is not insignificant."

RESTAURANTEUR IN KOLKATA

Asif Ahmed is collaborating with a few other organizations to prepare and deliver meals to several neighborhoods in Kolkata. Asif's restaurant chain is involved with NRAI (National Restaurant Association of India, Kolkata Chapter) and together they started this initiative of serving the needy when the lockdown began. Initially, they aimed at feeding 100 people daily and gradually his friends joined, and other organizations too got involved. Currently, they are feeding 15,000 people daily. "We are trying that while the lockdown continues, a one-time meal could be provided from our end. We are doing it in Kolkata now. However, NRAI branches are there in other cities also across the country. Every city, the organization is doing something or the other. Like Delhi, Bombay (Mumbai), Bangalore, people are joining hands to help others."

ON PEOPLE'S PARTICIPATION

"My friends are involved, and regular people of Kolkata have also come up. Then there are other organizations who want to get into this, and we are welcoming them because doing something like this alone on a large scale is difficult." They are relying on restaurants like Wow Momo for the kitchen space. "Depending on the staff count, we are collaborating with restaurant chains across the country or the local ones." There are six kitchens right now, and he confirms that two-three more are about to start.

For this initiative, a lot of supplies are needed, and most shops or markets do have not regular work hours. "From getting everything ready including groceries and other essentials to setting up the kitchens and preparing meals, we have to keep a lot in check. So, we are joining hands with whoever wants to get on board." To reach out to people, "we normally post on Facebook. I will send you that link, and the write-up which is there from where people can actually participate by donating money or whichever form they want. We are getting calls from various other cities as well. People are trying to reach out through me, and we are able to connect to those who need help now."

ON THE RELIEF WORK

"We are doing this with the help of Kolkata police. So, a lot of police stations, almost 20–25 police stations are already associated with us and helping us in the process of providing vehicles, collecting food, and distributing the same in localities across the city. Kolkata police are doing an excellent job in this. They are procuring food from our kitchens and providing it to the shelters where several daily wagers are staying. Apart from these shelters, we are providing food to a few other centers as and when we are getting connected with them. Mostly, these people are the daily wagers and people who are staying in slums and have no means to earn and feed their families. We are taking help of Kolkata police so they can reach out to areas and give tokens to residents. Accordingly they can come, maintain safe distances during distribution, and they can control the crowd because doing it individually again might be a very chaotic thing because the moment those people see our team coming with the packed food, they all want to throng and try to grab as much as they can. Therefore, we are routing through the police."

ON STAFF SAFETY AND OTHER PRECAUTIONS

"We are aware that there is a lot of fear as in people are not really wanting to come in contact. So, we are ensuring that staff are taking care of their safety. Each and every outlet that is participating – they are taking utmost care in this. They are using masks, sanitizers, and we are trying to keep the working area clean. When we are handling food, we are also trying to sanitize as much as possible."

"My whole day goes into this, and I hardly find time. I don't know whether it is lockdown or not. My entire team is involved in this. It seems even more hectic than a regular day at work." Ever since the lockdown was announced, Ahmed has never felt that industries have temporarily shut down. Rather, his days have become busier as he got involved in this initiative to do his bit in this moment. Ahmed feels this lockdown will continue for a long time, and they are looking forward to people's involvement in their relief projects. "We are trying our best to continue while the lockdown goes on. Therefore, we welcome more people's participation."

NOTES

1. For more on this term, please check: www.tandfonline.com/doi/abs/10.1300/J082v11n03_03?journalCode=wjhm20 (accessed May 5, 2020).
2. For more on Butalia's insights, please check: https://tribune.com.pk/story/124276/bringing-indias-transgenders-into-the-mainstream/ (accessed May 5, 2020).
3. Launched in 1995, the Mid-day Meal Scheme is a school meal program of the Indian government designed to better the nutritional standing of school-age children nationwide.

PART III

Southern Africa (Mozambique, South Africa and Zimbabwe)

CHAPTER SEVEN

Confronting State Authoritarianism: Civil Society and Community-Based Solidarity in Southern Africa

Boaventura Monjane

In southern Africa, measures taken by states and governments[1] to contain or delay the spread of Covid-19 are characterized by intensive militarization. Repressive state apparatus have been activated or intensified in most of the countries to enforce lockdown or State of Emergency regulations and monitor the movements of civilians. A critical aspect here is that the regulations prohibit the exercise of various economic activities practiced by many people in the so-called informal sector. The enforcement of the lockdown regulations has, therefore, been threatening the livelihoods of millions. The informal sector is predominant in southern Africa, mainly in the trade sector and is dominated by women.

In Zimbabwe, there were terrible incidences of police beating up and arresting street vendors, confiscating and destroying fresh vegetables and other foods of small-scale farmers who were selling at an open market. In Mozambique, the abusive behavior of a police officer, who slapped a disabled old man, was exposed through social media platforms by members of the public. In March (2020), South African police fired rubber bullets at shoppers queuing for food outside a supermarket in the city of Johannesburg.[2]

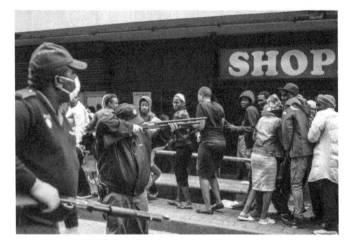

Figure 7.1   A South African policeman points his pump rifle to disperse a crowd of shoppers in Yeoville, Johannesburg, on March 28, 2020 while trying to enforce a safety distance outside a supermarket. (Photo by Marco Longari/AFP)

This chapter focuses on Mozambique, South Africa and Zimbabwe. The Mozambican President Filipe Jacinto Nyusi declared on March 30 the State of Emergency for 30 days and extended it for another month on April 30. The South African President Cyril Ramaphosa announced on March 23 that the country would be going into lockdown for 21 days, then extended the lockdown to the end of April. But on April 23, he announced an easing of the lockdown through a phased reopening of the economy, which began on May 1. Zimbabwe announced a 21-day national lockdown on March 30. On May 1, Zimbabwe's President Emmerson Mnangagwa extended the lockdown by two more weeks.

This chapter looks at responses from "below," based on interviews with activist leaders in civil society initiatives that emerged to articulate solidarity actions and monitor state actions in implementing the lockdown and State of Emergency. Paula Assubuji and Kelly Gillespie are both from C19 People's Coalition in South Africa. The coalition was born in March 2020, and includes 300 organizations from across civil society in all provinces, including community-based organizations, social movements, NGOs, research institutions and faith-based organizations – the broadest grouping of civil society that has come together to address the current crisis. We developed a Programme of Action (POA). Erika Mendes is from the Mozambican C-19 Civil Society Alliance, a broad collective of organizations, collectives and individuals who seek, in an articulate and organized way, to contribute to the construction of an active and inclusive citizenship, in the face of the Covid-19 world pandemic and the State of Emergency decreed in Mozambique. Erika also works for the NGO Justiça Ambiental. Jason Brickhill is from the Zimbabwe Covid-19 Support Hub, a group of Zimbabwean professionals and researchers in the diaspora and in Zimbabwe deeply concerned about the threat of the virus to Zimbabweans. Jason is a lawyer and Ph.D student in Oxford, UK.

From my conversation with these activist leaders, the following topics came to the fore: (1) anti-repression, (2) strengthening of civil society alliances, (3) diaspora solidarity, and (4) anti-xenophobic and regional solidarity. In the following sections, I provide the dialogue with these activist leaders, letting them speak in the first person. The last section brings some (un)concluding reflections for further debates.

ANTI-REPRESSION

> The harassment, beating, and rape of township residents and informal settlement dwellers by police and the army must stop.[3] (C19 People's Coalition Statement, April 2020)

When the lockdown was announced on March 23 in South Africa, more than 2,800 soldiers were deployed to assist the police with enforcing the lockdown regulations. In mid-April, South African President Cyril Ramaphosa announced that he had deployed an additional number of 73,180 members of the military[4] – almost all of the national army – allegedly to support the people and save lives: "This is a moment to be supportive to our people. I, therefore, order you to go out and execute this mission with great success,"[5] he said. Several cases of police (and army) abuse of power and brutality have been reported since the lockdown was decreed, especially in densely populated poor neighborhoods of South Africa, Zimbabwe and Mozambique.

As I write these lines, an activist from Botswana told me that – although not as visible as in South Africa and Zimbabwe – the police and the defense force are controlling roadblocks and enforcing lockdown regulations, using excessive violence towards people who allegedly break the law in a manner never seen before.

Mozambique is going through an armed conflict of alarming proportions, with insurgent groups operating in the minerals and gas rich northern province of Cabo Delgado. The Mozambican state has recently acknowledged that this is an external terrorist invasion. Mozambican President Filipe Nyusi has deployed the army to act "against" the terrorist insurgents. Civil society thinks this may be a pretext for the army to abuse its power and violate human and democratic rights of citizens.

The increased militarization and consequent reinforcement of authoritarianism as a pretext to fight the pandemic in these countries has triggered the formation of intersectoral civil society coalitions in several countries in the region. These coalitions are not only building alliances between various civil society organizations and groups in their countries, but also seeking to articulate with each other across borders.

We were very worried by the measures taken by the government to enforce the State of Emergency as we understood that it would further worsen the conditions of the majority of Mozambicans. These are people that work in the informal sector, most of them have to work every day to be able to put food on the table. So the State of Emergency might deteriorate the conditions of people that are already living in poverty, have been going hungry and are malnourished. (Erika Mendes, Mozambique, interview)

The state has also been very tough in its approach to the fight against Covid-19. The president of Mozambique said in an address to the nation that if citizens do not comply with the regulation the state would use force.[6] In Zimbabwe the scenario is no different:

The messages from the State are messages of threats. Threats of enforcement of the law, that you will be arrested if you break this regulation, rather than messages of solidarity. Zimbabwe State has normally been authoritarian. This will be aggravated now in this Covid-19 context. (Jason Brickhill, Zimbabwe, interview)

CIVIL SOCIETY ALLIANCES

With very few exceptions, civil society groups are not in the habit of working together on common agendas. This is true in Mozambique as it is in Zimbabwe and South Africa. For example, in South Africa, an attempt to articulate civil society groups from various sectors – such as the C19 People's Coalition, with more than 300 organizations – was attempted in the period following the abolition of apartheid. As Kelly G. explains,

There has been post-apartheid attempts at coalition building. None of them has really worked. Often they fall apart because there was not something specific to work on. What is most interesting about this coalition is that almost organically, out of the program of action, it is the organic emergence of working groups around particular issues. So there is a whole range of issues and in those working groups, some people have worked together before, but a lot of people haven't worked together before. And a lot of people haven't been compelled by a progressive vision of how this is in services of poor and working class communities. So there is something about the time of the crisis and the possibility that the coalition has afforded to have people to sit down and actually work together regardless of their differences. The kinds of relationships that have emerged out of that have been very important. (Interview, Kelly G., South Africa)

It has also been very common to see the segregation of struggles and movements among Mozambique civil society groups, which has long contributed to the segregated processes of resistance among social movements and activists. As Monjane and Bruna show,[7] "historically, urban-based struggles have had little dialogue with rural-based struggles. Trade unions have had little dialogue with peasant/agrarian organizations" and so on. It is therefore a novelty that in the C1-19 Civil Society Alliance there are almost 70 intersectorial organizations, including the largest – and first formed – trade union in Mozambique, the Sindicato dos Trabalhadores Moçambicanos (OTM, Mozambican Workers Union).

COMMUNITY-BASED SOLIDARITY

According to Elisio Macamo,

Africans have always responded to crises by appealing to their vibrant social safety nets for protection and action. This is not a romantic view of the continent. It is a pragmatic acknowledgement of the continent's real situation, one to which Africans have responded in resilient ways, even if at great human cost.[8]

As the author of the above quote rightly argues, lockdowns in most parts of the African continent "at least theoretically, weaken [those] safety nets by depriving individuals both of sources of livelihood as well as of opportunities for bonding." This thinker is certainly referring, but not exclusively, to the practice of Ubuntu, which in various communities in southern Africa is expressed by individuals and groups providing social and community service to the others. Ubuntu is a Nguni Bantu term meaning "humanity." It is often translated as "I am because we are" or "humanity towards others."

The solidarity actions underway in southern Africa aim precisely to reinforce this idea, even in situations where the state criminalizes it. In the Western Cape province of South Africa, a collective of women were doing community kitchen work, distributing hot food to hungry people in their community. Police intervened and beat them up for doing an activity that was allegedly prohibited under the lockdown. The collective approached the C19 People's Coalition. The coalition approached a social justice lawyer who helped to organize a meeting with the prevention police commissioner. As a result of that meeting, not only was this women's collective allowed to resume the community kitchen, but it was also regulated that this solidarity activity is allowed throughout the Western Cape province.

That is a very grounded example of offering solidarity and resources and skills to a particular community kitchen and a particular neighborhood and facilitating a conversation with law enforcement can have an anti-repressive consequence. And then we as a coalition began to mobilize for that in other regions. (Interview, Kelly Gillespie, South Africa)

A large number of community-based solidarity initiatives, mainly concerned with the distribution of food, face masks and other essential items – including solidarity pricing in community markets – to vulnerable groups and working class people, are taking place around southern Africa.

DIASPORA INTERVENTIONS

The Zimbabwean and Mozambican diaspora also mobilized to provide solidarity with communities in their home countries. The support from citizens of these countries living abroad to their families is not a new practice. For instance, it is estimated that between 2 and 3 million Zimbabwean citizens living abroad send, all together, millions of dollars in remittances per year. But Covid-19 brings a different sort of sensitivity. The Zimbabwe Covid-19 Support Hug was founded with a pretty new spirit:

We are a group of Zimbabwean professionals and researchers in the diaspora and in Zimbabwe. We created this project as a way to support efforts of Government,

civil society and communities in Zimbabwe to respond
to the virus (Interview, Jason Brickhill)

This "hub" has been mobilizing in solidarity to support
and amplify local initiatives and capacity with medical
equipment, testing kits, food items and other type of
donations.

The "hub" has also been holding live Q&A sessions
where doctors (both in Zimbabwe and abroad) respond
to questions. "We have been having hundreds of people
asking questions about how to stay safe, about testing, the
use of masks. It is about bringing together different skills
and energy in the community to work together to respond
to the pandemic," said Brickhill. Together with medical
students in Zimbabwe the "hub" has been able to translate
Covid-19 information into Shona, Ndebele and Kalanga
(Bantu languages spoken by millions of Zimbabweans).

Some initiatives by the Mozambican diaspora have also
been promoting fundraising campaigns. Recently a group
of diaspora organizations launched a campaign called
"Food for Rural Mozambique," mobilizing the diaspora
mainly in Europe and the US to support Mozambique.
There was also a webinar[9] in which prominent Mozambican academics and a congress woman representing the
Mozambican diaspora in Europe and the rest of the world
discussed how the country could overcome the crisis and
what role the Mozambican diaspora could play in the
process.

How are these efforts different to charity? Jason Brickhill explains the difference:

There are few important principles that, at least for us, distinguish solidarity from charity. For us, part of it is just personal that we are all connected with our communities and families. At the political level for us it is important that we are *supporting* and not *supplanting* [emphasis added] local community efforts. We are promoting the actions of people that are in the front line in the ground. And [also] building networks, reaching out to different groups, communities and organizations.

ANTI-XENOPHOBIA AND REGIONAL SOLIDARITY

South Africa is "home" for millions of migrant people, especially from neighboring countries such as Zimbabwe, Mozambique and Malawi.[10] This is due to its economy, which is historically dependent on immigrant labor, as well as the geopolitical position South Africa occupies. South Africa is the second largest African economy after Nigeria and has a GDP of $349.3 billion. Migrants of these countries are mostly employed in the food, agriculture and mining sectors. A huge number of them are, however, in the so-called informal sector. These people have been largely left behind by South African government support actions – as they generally are under normal circumstances.

Not surprisingly, 23,000 Mozambicans crossed the Lebombo/Ressano Garcia border[11] alone the day before the confinement announced by President Cyril Ramaphosa came into effect.[12] They knew they would be victims of social exclusion, so they ran away from starvation and xenophobia. The South African government has not set a good example in discouraging xenophobia. In his public announcements, President Cyril Ramaphosa insists on addressing the public as fellow "South Africans" in a country with millions of non-national citizens. Very recently, the South African Minister of Finance, Tito Titus Mboweni, said on public TV that:

> Any new establishment wanting to reopen [after the lockdown] must have a new labour market policy which priorities South Africans ... That is the new economy we are talking about. People who want to approach banks or government for funding and so on must demonstrate that they have a Labour market and employment policy that favour South Africans.[13]

Under the pretext of avoiding the importation of coronavirus into the country, the South African government announced the construction of a fence on the Beitbridge border between South Africa and Zimbabwe, costing South Africans and migrant workers in the country R37 million (about $2 million).[14] It is in this context that a regional solidarity working group was created in the South African C19 People's Coalition.

Paula Assubuji, who also works for the Heinrich Boell Foundation South Africa, explains more:

> When we were creating the coalition we paused to think of how does one build solidarity that goes beyond the borders of South Africa. Because it was obvious that this was a global crisis and it was obvious that the issues would pretty much be similar, although in different

contexts, in other societies and the closing down of South African borders would have a very strong impact in the region. So we came up with the idea of building a regional solidarity network that goes beyond South Africa geographical boarders. So, the coalition felt that there was a need to reach out to similar networks and initiatives, also in terms of linking the struggles because the struggles are intertwined to each other.

The C19-People's Coalition sent a letter on May 13 to South Africa's president Ramaphosa, who is also the chairperson of the African Union, reminding him that he has "committed to deepening unity across the Continent, mainstreaming the needs of women, and championing the position of Africa globally. And yet, in all of the

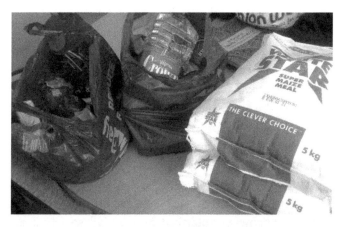

Figure 7.2   Food parcels by the People Against Suffering, Oppression and Poverty (PASSOP) to LGBT people, disabled refugees and asylum seekers during the national lockdown in April, Cape Town, South Africa. (Photo by Victor Chikalogwe|PASSOP)

public statements communicating South Africa's efforts to fight Covid-19 [he has] excluded migrants, refugees, and asylum seekers living in this country. The consistent lack of recognition fuels xenophobic attitudes and intensifies the human and economic toll of Covid-19. It is also inconsistent with the crisis of the times; the preamble of the South African constitution and your role as the AU chair," reads the letter.[15]

CONCLUSION

The civil society networks that are emerging around Covid-19 are not only focused on the pandemic. They are "seizing the opportunity" to radicalize demands and thus push for a restructuring in the balance of forces between the state, capital and society. And as Chuma Mgcoyi, a South African permaculture practitioner, says,

> solidarity is a must. We don't have a choice. No one knows actually what will happen tomorrow and who will need whom. So, it is a matter of activating Ubuntu and care for each other, regardless of proximity, borders or race. We are all in this. (Interview, Chuma Mgcoyi, South Africa)

This seems to be exactly the case. The position papers and various statements published by the civil society coalitions, mainly in Mozambique and South Africa, demand a transformation of society that goes beyond fighting the pandemic:

As soon as possible, it is equally urgent that we rethink the path we are setting out on, and begin to move towards sustainable social, economic and human development. Civil society must be seen as playing a key role in building active citizenship, for all. This is the challenge – and also the opportunity – that the Covid-19 pandemic presents us with.[16]

NOTES

1. www.dailymail.co.uk/news/article-8162889/Police-South-Africa-fire-RUBBER-BULLETS-hundreds-shoppers.html (accessed May 19, 2020).
2. Ibid.
3. https://c19peoplescoalition.org.za/statement-bread-not-bullets/ (accessed April 28, 2020).
4. www.sabcnews.com/sabcnews/ramaphosa-deploys-additional-73-000-soldiers/ (accessed May 4, 2020).
5. www.youtube.com/watch?v=cc1AVwB8H28&feature=emb_title (accessed May 2, 2020).
6. https://web.facebook.com/NyusiConfioemti/videos/72144 6258594262/ (accessed May 8, 2020).
7. www.tandfonline.com/doi/full/10.1080/03066150.2019.16 71357 (accessed April 29, 2020).
8. Elisio Macamo, Mozambican scholar and sociologist: www.coronatimes.net/normality-risk-african-european-responses/ (accessed May 19, 2020).
9. www.youtube.com/watch?v=PYfKaWJEFOg&feature=youtu.be (accessed April 20, 2020).
10. https://naijaquest.com/largest-economies-in-africa/ (accessed April 28, 2020).
11. This is the main and most strategic border between Mozambique and South Africa. It is situated between the city of Komatipoort in Mpumalanga province (South Africa) and

the municipality of Ressano Garcia in Maputo province (Mozambique).

12. https://allafrica.com/stories/202003270901.html (accessed April 30, 2020).

13. SABC News, "SA Lockdown: Minister Mboweni Briefs the Media on Economic Measures," April 25, 2020,

14. www.thesouthafrican.com/news/beitbridge-border-fence-coronavirus/ (accessed May 19, 2020).

15. The letter is available here: https://c19peoplescoalition.org.za/open-letter-to-president-ramaphosa-end-state-led-xen-ophobia-now/ (accessed May 19, 2020).

16. https://aliancac19.wordpress.com/ (accessed April 18, 2020).

PART IV

Europe (Portugal, Greece, Italy and the UK)

CHAPTER EIGHT

On Intersectional Solidarity in Portugal

Laís Gomes Duarte and Raquel Lima

I will keep writing about these intersections as a writer and a teacher, as a black woman, as a bad feminist, until I no longer feel like what I want is impossible. I no longer want to believe that these problems are too complex for us to make sense of them. (Roxane Gay, "Bad Feminist")

INTRODUCTION

The State of Emergency in response to the Covid-19 pandemic was declared by the Portuguese government on March 18, 2020 and scheduled to last for 15 days. It was subsequently renewed twice and on May 2, Prime Minister Antonio Costa declared the country had entered "the state of calamity." The State of Emergency demanded compulsory confinement at home, with the exception of jobs considered essential for the country's health and economy. One of the curious aspects of the decree was the suspension of the right of resistance, preventing any and all acts of active or passive resistance to orders issued by the public authorities in execution of the emergency state. This proposal raised a series of inconsistencies and concerns. Activist groups from all over the country inquired about the conditions of vulnerable communities – such as undocumented immigrants, unhoused, racialized people and informal market workers. As our interviewees have noted, black and Romani Portuguese communities have been subject to historically structured inequalities and social injustices, and their survival and social reproduction are exactly based on the forms of resistance (and solidarity) that the State of Emergency decree had criminalized.

Activists from the Anti-Racist Campaign for Immediate Support of Coimbra have asked:

As we work with families in the Roma community of 15 people living in 3 bedroom apartments, we wondered how can people maintain social distancing or stay at home and their movements be monitored, if they live off what they can earn while on the street? If they don't have savings, nor access to income replacements, would staying at home mean risking their main sources of income during this process? Even if the State introduces wage substitution and social security support subsidies, how will this work for people who do undeclared informal work? If confinement is connected with an isolation, testing and treatment strategy, what does confinement mean where there is no such strategy? Thinking about authoritarianism, would it be possible for the military and police to actually fulfill their role of public security and protection in a context in which black and Roma people have been dehumanized and violated historically by the State and capital?[1]

Understanding what solidarity can mean in this context implies reflecting on the different connotations and appropriations of the term throughout the country's history, whether through dominant narratives or underground discourses. During the colonial period solidarity rhetoric was used in a paternalistic sense by the Salazar-Caetano dictatorship to legitimize colonial occupation and domination of African colonies, which according to the regime needed to be saved from inherent savagery, moral and cultural inferiority by civilized, morally and culturally superior people, like the Portuguese. From 1961 onwards, when the first revolutionary winds of the anti-colonial struggle were blown from Guinea-Bissau, Cape Verde, Angola, Mozambique and São Tomé e Príncipe in Africa, anti-colonial networks that joined forces to fight for a liberated Africa gave solidarity a new symbol to uphold. Because of initiatives such as the clandestine revolutionary party PAIGC (African Party for the Independence of Guinea Bissau and Cape Verde) solidarity had become from that point forward a symbol of the anti-colonial struggle. From 1986 onwards, when Portugal joined the European Union (EU), solidarity was portrayed as a cornerstone value of the bloc and used as justification for the financial aid that the EU provided to the struggling economies of members like Portugal, Italy, Greece and Spain. Today, it is for and from the margins of Portuguese society that solidarity has once again gained a counter-hegemonic usage as our interviews show.

Although Portugal stands out in the international press for its success in stopping the spread of coronavirus, for the disciplined way in which its inhabitants have fulfilled social isolation, many of the activists interviewed in this chapter are focused on recognizing at whose expense this success has been achieved. For these activists, doing solidarity work means doing what the state does not do in the margins of society. In the words of one of our interviewees, Claudia Cambraia from Projeto Nzinga: "To be in solidarity is to place oneself in the shoes of another, it's to perceive one's lack of access to the means of survival, it's to keep in mind social inequities."

This meaning is carried in the work of the people and organizations interviewed, chosen considering the actions, groups and associations with which we had a relationship and/or were involved. We made an effort to encompass initiatives that were not located in a single city, thus we gathered interviews from Lisbon, Coimbra and Oporto. The interviewees' perspectives on solidarity and mutual support for building a more just society led us to understand the importance which they give, through their actions, to the intersections, connections and partnerships between different people and different social causes, which in turn led us to inquire about the configurations that intersectionality gains when put into practice. We learned to see the process of gradually increased commitment through diverse struggles as a process of intersectional solidarity. Three of the cases – DialogAR Network, the Anti-Racist Campaign for Immediate Support of Coimbra and the Popular Network for Mutual Support of Oporto – are collectives that existed in a pre-pandemic world and joined forces in the wake of the Covid-19 crisis. Their collaboration shows that the meaning that solidarity gained during the anti-colonial wars still exists in this so-called postcolonial country.

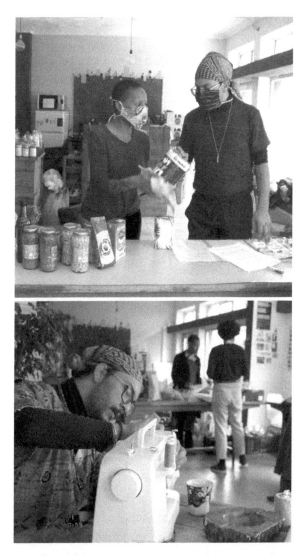

Figures 8.1. and 8.2 Taken in the context of the Popular Network for Mutual Support in Oporto, by one of the activists. (Photo courtesy of Dori Nigro/NARP)

INTERVIEWS

We counted on the generous help of a number of activists associated with the initiatives described below, all promoting their work through social media without political party or union support. In most cases, they speak in the first-person plural, respecting the collective voice that represents the initiatives. We asked if they could share with us how they were feeling, what they had been doing and what kind of future they imagined and hoped for in a post-pandemic world. The interviews were open to other possible reflections on this topic.

Plataforma Geni (Lisboa)

An autonomous online platform made for and by immigrant women to promote women's empowerment and rights. During the pandemic, they have formed a solidarity network by inviting immigrant women to ask for and to offer psychological social, and material support.

We are, like most people, concerned and apprehensive about the future, mainly because we have contact with many women in situations of social vulnerability and with complex problems. But we are calm and reasonable at the moment, seeking to inform ourselves and following recommendations of the Portuguese government. We have been working firmly and together while trying to help women who come to us for help through Plataforma Geni, which usually organizes instructional discussion groups to help immigrant women learn and practice a second language. Our goal is to help women learn more about their rights and empower themselves; all classes are organized with themes regarding gender equality. In addition, we hold a feminist conversation circle to connect new insights and ideas by bringing together several women to discuss topics that are dear to us. In all projects, we see women creating bonds and friendships with each other. This leaves us immensely grateful and happy, motivating us to continue and develop other projects. For instance, we are currently impressed by the willingness of women volunteering to help one another in the pandemic. We've created a solidarity network to support Brazilian immigrant women in Portugal. We did not expect that so many people would be available to help. Through a form shared on our social networks, women can ask for and offer psychological, social, and material support. All appointments are made online by women professionally trained in the services offered. In the case of women who didn't have food available we were able to help by collecting monetary donations and redistributing it to those who needed it. We have seen that women want to help. We have managed to bring these women together and direct help to those who need it most. We believe that the pandemic will bring reflections on how we use our time, on forms of consumption and on our personal and social relationships. The solidarity network formed through the Plataforma Geni showed us how much we can do and that we have the strength to collaborate. This is rich. After the pandemic we hope that people will look at the collective and rethink their social practices, just as we have been rethinking ours. We imagine and hope for a more equitable, just and conscientious future.

Grupo Educar (Lisboa)

A collective formed by anti-racist educators to develop methodologies for anti-racist education based on the Portuguese reality. Through workshops they gather educators online and in physical spaces to build ways to combat everyday structural racism. During the pandemic, they united efforts with three other collectives, the Kazumba Association, the European Support Network for Brazilian Victims of Domestic Violence and Together 2 Change, to create the DialogAR Network – offering psychological and emotional support, legal advice, and artistic, mindfulness and language instruction for immigrant families.

While searching for what to do in this context – as we already imagined that to quarantine would be impossible for so many and would put all of us at other risks, we believed that it would be important and possible to create a mutual-aid and mental health support network to offer what we called "solidary listening," and to offer legal advice by counting on the help of specialized professionals, by focusing on the needs of immigrants and workers, and by fundraising to redistribute money and pantry supplies. We used social media to distribute a virtual public forum that allowed us to pair those willing to offer free counselling and legal advice with people in need of these services. The confinement promoted by the quarantine made us think about family relationships through reports of domestic violence, involving couples, elderly people and children. So we organized a weekly program to entertain and reassure everyone through social media. We offered dance classes for children, storytelling focusing on Afro-Brazilian and Afrocentric content, guided meditation, Italian language courses, virtual dinner parties, know your rights info sessions, and thematic discussion groups. This autonomous, collective, unpaid and non-profit initiative helped us to take care of ourselves and of those around us. Recognizing our limitations and privileges, we found an alternative form of movement. We believe that solidarity strengthens ties. The DialogAR Network is a tool that helped us to portray the countless violations of fundamental rights that existed before the pandemic but which were "difficult to demonstrate." We see a clear picture of the countless structural and institutional barriers reported by immigrants in their integration path and the absence of immediate government measures to support these groups. There is a willingness from everyone to continue with the DialogAR Network after the quarantine is over, since this return to "normalcy" tends to generate even more or newer imbalances. We are looking for formats and ways to continue. We believe that the worst is yet to come. For this reason we believe that mutual-aid networks and mental health support will continue to be essential to the survival of all.

Associação Social Recreativa Cultural Cigana de Coimbra (Coimbra)

A private institution of social solidarity serving the community of Planalto do Ingote in Coimbra, in the socio-cultural mediation between institutions and the mixed community. We interviewed activist Osvaldo Grilo who's been collaborating with Núcleo Antirracista de Coimbra (NAC) and Projeto Nzinga in the scope of the Anti-Racist Campaign for Immediate Support of Coimbra.

With the Covid-19 pandemic a new scenario was established, making contact with people from the Roma community more difficult, both due to rules of social distancing and to their lack of access to mobile cell phones and internet, lack of funds for making phone calls and fear of contamination by the coronavirus. The work routine of Roma people has undergone changes, since our main work activity is trade in fairs or homes, and provision of seasonal services. With the state of emergency, we were prevented from exercising our functions and there was no government policy to meet the demand of this social group, which has led to hunger, panic, disorientation and worsening of our mental health. Added to this the Roma community lacks information about how coronavirus contamination occurs, which can affect our ability to protect ourselves against the disease, thus making us more susceptible to contagion. The health crisis has given us the task of expanding our solidarity networks to obtain more support for Roma people. The contact with Núcleo Antirracista de Coimbra (NAC) was a way to move forward with our purposes of seeking immediate support. Thus, we use social networks to give more visibility to our cause in an attempt to raise awareness and convert this awareness into food for Roma families. Our opportunity to establish a connection with the Projeto Nzinga and NAC reiterated our vision of how we, racialized people, experience in daily life a situation permeated by racism, xenophobia and anti-gypsyism. However, exchanging ideas and joint actions, we can better understand the different realities and prepare ourselves for our community aid actions that tend to last for a long time.

Projeto Nzinga (Coimbra)

A project for social intervention to combat social exclusion, gender and racial inequality through the reclamation of African and Afro-descendant culture.

From March 2020, with the declaration by the WHO of the Covid-19 pandemic (11/03) and State of Emergency in Portugal (18/03), there was a significant change in the request for support. Previously supported families activated others, who started to contact the Projeto Nzinga, with requests for assistance, which we responded to through a friendship network, informally. After that, members of NAC contacted us in order to strengthen ties and we became a part of the Anti-Racist Campaign for Immediate Support of Coimbra. We connect to this campaign, by identifying ourselves with the supported women, because, in addition to empathy, our members identify as black women, immigrants, mothers that originated from a "popular" social class and have always been participating in projects with the purpose of expanding the citizenship for all, so social confinement did not prevent my/our solidarity action.

On the contrary, with agility, we reevaluated the actions and together we formed a collaborative network, we built new social organization models, thus increasing the use of social media – Facebook and electronic newsletters, for example – to enable collaborations for black women and their families, and we were successful. Despite this, we need to reflect on people in situations of social vulnerability in times of crisis, respecting their autonomy and decisions, without victimizing them. In my understanding, charity is linked to an unequal, impersonal relationship, the donation from people with possessions to the poorest, the offering of "crumbs," in some cases, in search of social prestige. Assistentialism, on the other hand, is related to institutional support for groups in need in the long term, in which people are seen as "eternally dependent on the State." In turn, being solidarity is putting yourself in the other person's shoes, realizing his/her lack of access to means of survival, for example, with social inequalities in mind. Solidarity aid can take different forms, such as food support, the formation of bonds of friendship and the monitoring of families until the crisis is overcome.

Popular Network for Mutual Support (Porto)

Born out of a joint effort between four grassroots organizations this group has been active since March 19, organizing collective solidarity actions that respond to vital community needs amplified by the Covid-19 crisis.

Our actions are aimed at anyone who is affected by the pandemic, without placing the bureaucratic obstacles found in the institutional channels. In order to safeguard everyone's care and well-being, we have created a hygiene and safety protocol applied to all moments of personal contact. Logistical support has been another strategy. We contacted those who need help with shopping, garbage collection or walking animals to connect them with people willing to offer these services. We have disseminated critical information on health, migration, labor rights, gender-based violence, social security, housing, sex work, collective care and mutual support, both through social media and by posting information on physical spaces. We've also created a hotline so that people can ask questions on health or ask for support if they feel anxious or worried because of this situation. One of our concerns from the beginning was to build a network of mutual support and not an aid project. The network is based on solidarity and not on charity. This is important to us as we criticize charity because we see it as a washing of the image and conscience of those who benefit from social inequalities and who have no interest in questioning them, consciously or unconsciously. Thus, the Popular Network for Mutual Support is driven by equally precarious bodies that seek to dismantle power relations, bureaucratic control and moralizing discourses, recognizing the experiences (often of systemic marginalization) of those who access it. To this end, we use methods such as informal communication and intentional safe and caring spaces. This initiative is generated from the ground up, rooted in horizontality and self-management, and it is born from the cooperation of collectives that share political affinities and already had direct-action projects in place to resist the current system in a pre-pandemic world.

CONCLUSION

When we talk about intersectional solidarity, we see examples of solidarity and mutual aid about which our interviewees speak as powerful *praxis*, which means putting theory into practice and practice into theory. In that sense we chose to interview people involved in campaigns developed by different groups, associations and collectives that met on a common task, allowing them to understand the social inequalities that permeate the dynamic structure in which they live. As the activists from the Popular Network for Mutual Support mentioned: "What the pandemic makes evident immediately is that the current economic and social system is based on a structure of patriarchal, racist and classist exploitation, which causes inequalities that the pandemic has only exacerbated. The current system operates from a hierarchy of bodies, defining those who have access to the sphere of living and those who are marked as precarious, disposable and killable. In our political action, we seek to contemplate the way in which different systems of oppression intersect and legitimize each other, to question and deconstruct the operations of these systems at a macropolitical and micropolitical level, to unveil the relationships between power/privilege/oppression, to recognize the different places speaking and listening, as well as thinking and acting for the construction of dialogues, affinities and collective action with a view to social transformation."

The experiences of interviewing and writing this chapter have taught us that to develop a new vision of intersectional solidarity that is not beholden to the hegemonic models of the past, but inspired by local struggles and achieves the remaking of humanism, seems to be one of the most crucial intellectual and political tasks of our time.

NOTE

1. From the podcast Radio Gabriela: https://soundcloud.com/user-317333437/entrevista_nac_radiogabriela (accessed May 1, 2020).

CHAPTER NINE

Solidarity Flourishes Under Lockdown in Italy

Eleanor Finley

And if I die as a partisan
You must bury me
And you must bury me up there on the mountain
Under the shade of a beautiful flower.

("Bella, Ciao!" – anonymous)

The deadly outbreak of Covid-19 in Italy marked a turning point in global conversation about the pandemic. Many Westerners found it easy to dismiss the threat as something foreign when the disease struck China during the months of January and February. News of the outbreak in Italy, a relatively wealthy country with a celebrated healthcare system, was a sobering revelation. This shock was compounded by the fact that Lombardy – the fashion capital and the country's wealthiest region – was the epicenter. If a Covid-19 epidemic could happen in Lombardy, it could happen anywhere.

By Tuesday, March 9, Prime Minister Giuseppe Conte declared the entire country a "red zone." Citizens were confined to their homes unless permitted by police via "self-certification" (*autocertificazione*). All travel and leisure ceased as church bells sang to deserted streets. Every night at 6 pm, the Protezione Civile, the state-run agency tasked with managing the crisis, announced staggering numbers of new infections and deaths.

The following interviews present five different perspectives on the pandemic lockdown and mutual aid projects in Northern Italy. Under normal circumstances, it is almost impossible to prevent Italians from being close to each other. But, as these voices demonstrate, it takes even more to keep them from acting in solidarity with their community. And sometimes, as one interviewee put it, "being in solidarity means being far away from each other."

That solidarity is elevated to the next level via the coordinated efforts of social centers and community groups such the Brigata Lena-Modotti ["Lena-Modotti Brigade] in Milan and Don't Panic – Organizziamoci!" [Don't Panic – Let's Organize!] in Bologna. From food collection and delivery to digital activism, call centers, and even pet sitting – individuals and organizations are working hard to support each other via formal and informal networks of mutual aid. These interviews were conducted in a mix of Italian and English languages and have been edited for length and clarity.

ZOE

Zoe is a high school student and Kurdish solidarity activist living in the Northeastern city of Genova. Her mother is an activist and a nurse on the frontline of the coronavirus struggle. I get in touch with Zoe when she asks me to

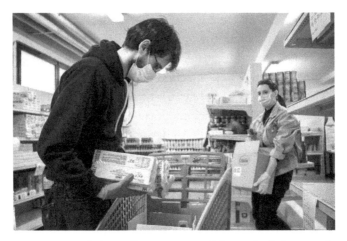

Figure 9.1 Solidarity Shopping – Don't Panic: Let's Organize! volunteers pick up food at the local food bank for distribution. Their campaign now feeds over 450 families. (Photo by Giulio Di Meo)

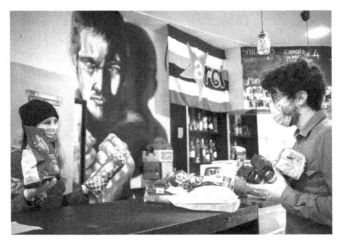

Figure 9.2 Don't Panic: Let's Organize! volunteers organize food like bread, flour and tuna fish for distribution at Ritmo Lento. (Photo by Giulio Di Meo)

participate in a march to honor the one-year anniversary of the death of Lorenzo "Orso" [Bear] Tekosher, an Italian socialist killed in the war against ISIS in Northern Syria. Although Italy had gone under full lockdown, Zoe didn't give up on honoring Lorenzo. She and her companions organized a flash mob at the windows to sing the Italian leftist anthem "Bella Ciao" while waving red, yellow and green handkerchiefs – the colors of Kurdish independence. The action was captured and broadcast via Florence independent radio and shared on social media. Ten days later, dozens of Kurdish musicians posted their own digital performance of "Bella Ciao" in the Kurdish language to show their solidarity with Italians.

What has been your experience so far with the Covid-19 outbreak in Italy?
It's a strange and difficult situation. My mom must go to work every day and now she works in a retirement home. Because there aren't many spaces in the hospital, they must isolate and treat Covid patients within the facility. I haven't been out for two months because of the quarantine. And I am also working to keep and feed the animals of people who are in the hospital, so I have many animals in my home right now. Usually, when I'm at home, I'm drawing or reading books. I must do online school too.

So, you are alone when your mother is working?
Yes, I am alone. I have a half-sister, but she lives in another part of the city so I can't see her at this moment. But I have the animals. I love animals. I'm a vegetarian.

Can you say more about that?

Yes, I have seven dogs – little dogs. I have two birds, two rabbits, and two parakeets. I get up and feed them every morning. We have a very big home, so they can walk around and enjoy themselves. They don't make any problems.

You are also working on mutual aid projects in Genoa right now?

Yes, I work on a fundraising project on Kurdistan and Rojava. I am carrying out this project with three companions. There are a lot of people that draw in Kurdistan. We do an exhibition with these drawings and then collect the money for the Kurdish Red Crescent.

How did you become involved with this project?

My mom has spoken to me about Kurdistan since I was very young. I decided to do this project with my friends. We are active in politics and for the planet as well. I also am involved with Fridays for the Future and Extinction Rebellion. The other young people from Fridays for the Future do similar activities, helping people who don't have a home or helping them with food and drink.

What is the Extinction Rebellion project doing now?

We are doing online strikes for climate change and for ecological issues. Usually, we do video calls to discuss the important arguments, but we organized this demonstration online. We make signs, we photograph the signs, and send the photos around on all of the social media platforms.

How has Kurdish solidarity activism changed after the pandemic?
I imagine that in Kurdistan they are really in difficulty in regard to this situation. In our situation we have a health system that is organized well enough, but I imagine they have a really hard job and need solidarity demonstrated in this moment. We must demonstrate it then. I work with my companions and we write to people who live in other countries, like Kurdistan, USA, or England. It's very important. Above everything else, during this moment, we need to demonstrate all of our solidarity. It doesn't really matter with which population we are demonstrating. It is enough that we are showing the solidarity from the one with the other because it's hard. These times are truly hard.

What do young people want for the future?
I think that the pandemic serves to show our shortcomings and we must adapt and listen to its teaching. We need a drastic change to our lives. We hope for a better world and better people. We hope that things will really change from how they are going now. We hope that people can be more in solidarity with each other and, certainly, we hope for things to get better.

EMILY

Emily is a 33-year-old law student who has lived her life in the city of Bologna in Northern Italy. She is also a city councillor representing the municipalist platform Coalizione Civica. Emilia Romagna is the second worst hit region by Covid-19. As a municipalist city councillor,

Emily had a unique role to play in Bologna's solidarity network, Don't Panic: Organizziamoci! [We Organize Ourselves!]. Don't Panic is a coalition project comprised of over 40 organizations – from anarchist trade unions to religious groups. The project is based in a social and political center, Ritmo Lento [Slow Rhythm]. Ritmo Lento is associated with a national network called Circolo Arci [the Arci Network]. It is a bar and cafe, as well as a meeting and assembly space that is occasionally converted into a co-working arrangement. Today, it is the central hub of Don't Panic's campaign "Spesa Solidale" [Solidarity Shopping] to bring food to the vulnerable.

> The first days of lockdown hit us hard. We're assembly animals. We're used to meeting and discussing and seeing each other all the time. It felt very strange to all of a sudden be at home and feeling unable to accomplish anything except work.
>
> We and Ritmo Lento are often working together on different issues, so it came naturally to collaborate on first response. What worked about this project was that instead of launching our own little campaign as Coalizione Civica or Ritmo Lento doing the same thing, we joined forces to make the most horizontal campaign possible so that maybe other associations will join.
>
> What I did as a city councillor was to call different people who work in city hall. Even though I am on the opposition, I explained that we really want to do whatever we can to help. The first days were tricky because obviously with the lockdown, you couldn't exit your house without a good reason. Even volunteering

wasn't covered. La Croce Rossa [the Red Cross] was trying not to give the message that you could just go out and help. So, we had to reach out to the city hall and ask if they could authorize us.

City hall gave us a first few tasks that we could do without any particular insurance. Right now, that's the important thing: insurance [to prevent accidents and lawsuits]. They said, "Right now our food banks are empty; we're running out of food. If you can collect food without having physical contact with people and just leave the food on people's doorstep, you won't need any particular insurance." So, that's something we started doing right away and we continue to do food bank runs every other day.

Now, many other projects and associations have started to join the Don't Panic! process and each is bringing their own spirit. Today, we launched a psycho-logical help phone line with different psychologists who have joined the campaign. There's also an info line for people who are having a hard time on their job site right now because maybe they are being forced to go to work even though there are positive cases among their co-workers, that sort of situation.

What does it feel like to do these pickups?
It literally feels like Ferragosto [a major Italian holiday on August 15], like a desert. Bologna is not close to the sea, so it gets very muggy in the summer. The 15th of August is the day when there is no one around at all and everything is shut down. It feels like we are stuck in that limbo except that there's no joy. The air is tense. You feel it when you go out. There are not a lot of people smiling;

everyone is very direct and going about their business. It's strange. Everything is just empty.

Do you feel like there are new possibilities opened up by this mutual aid collaboration?
The fact that there are so many different associations collaborating took me by surprise. For example, we have five or six LGBT organizations. Half of them are more collaborative with [government] institutions and another half – they don't even want to recognize them. To see these groups coming together and working – that surprised me. There are also associations in this which are more religious-oriented. Then there are sex worker organizations too. It's cool to see that variety. I wasn't expecting it and I hope it can be a chance to see that very different groups can work together if there is a common goal.

But I wonder if it wasn't for this kind of emergency, this urgency to get together and help each other – if these very diverse groups of people would be working together. I hope that's a chance to deepen that relationship and that bond. Groups that are skeptical of working together may discover that they *can* work well together and because they in fact have done so already.

Do you think these new forms of solidarity can persist after the crisis is over?
I don't think it'll be easy. The driving force [of this initiative] is the fact that this is an extraordinary time and people need to stick together. But we should try to keep this relationship going. It's not as if the quarantine finishes and we all go back to our normal lives,

the social and economic aftermath of this is going to be very long. We have to think that this mutual aid is going to be here for the long run.

It goes together with the fact that this system we have been living with has been shattered a bit. If this isn't a wake-up call on capitalism, what is? If we're living in a world where you're not allowed to stop for even two weeks or a month or *everything* falls apart, that must raise some questions. It's very interesting to see that now people are really advocating for a public health system or more funding in education and in research. *Patrimoniale* [graduated income taxing] has come up again in the debate.

What is the overarching lesson in all of this about care?
In Italy, care is heavily assigned to women – not just of children, but also of our elderly. That's something people are starting to understand and appreciate more. It needs to be evened out. Second, we need to invest in care. By "care" I also mean prevention. What progressive healthcare workers are trying to advocate for is searching for your patients in the community – to go and find them and test them *before* they degenerate into being seriously ill. We need to be taking care of people much earlier on. It's more sustainable economically and of course people live better that way. They get less sick. Yesterday was World Health Day and there were a lot of different experts advocating for this in Italy as well as all over the world. I find that perspective very important.

FRANCESCO

Francesco (32 years old) is a longtime activist and a dedicated member of the municipalist platform Coalizione Civica. Although he normally lives in Bologna, he is spending the lockdown with his father in his home in Morino, a small town outside of Rome. Francesco is a volunteer with Protezione Civile, the state-run organization responsible for providing aid and ensuring compliance with the special health and social distancing precautions. His experience provides a glimpse into the lives of tens of thousands of volunteers throughout every region of Italy.

Being a volunteer for the Protezione Civile means that every day is different. I don't do too much direct interventions like being on the front line, I help more on the bureaucratic side. But sometimes I do go out with them in their cars.

Some days, there's nothing to do, they just need to surveil and be ready. There are days where there are a lot of things to do. Sometimes getting ready for situations like going to get medicines for people that need it or assistance to people that have contracted the virus. I don't do that. I don't even get close to that. But mostly the mood of the team, which is all the people that live around here … they feel it every time they hear there are more positive cases of the virus, or if there is an increase of one or two in the death toll in Marino. They take it far more personally than I do. It's a small community, so everyone knows each other.

Regarding the relationship with the other volunteers of the Protezione Civile and as well with people you meet, civilians – ordinary people – on the one hand, I am very surprised as to how people are able to be resilient. I see a lot of capacity to go on and be of mutual help, of expressing solidarity with your neighbor. Especially in Italy and individualistic and sometimes closed-minded, racist, and identitarian behaviors are highlighted by media. It gives you an idea of a wild society out there, a very depressing, hopeless Hobbes-like state of nature, *uomini lupus* [man wolf]. That's not the case as soon as you get in touch with what's out there.

You see a lot of solidarity around. My hope is that we are able to thrive on that in order to build something. After this is over, to be able to say, remember what happened? Remember who you were supported by? It was your neighbor. So hopefully we can rebuild that sense of collective identity – positive collective identity, not negative, like the Right does. Positive in the sense that it builds on some common ground and that common ground is solidarity and mutual aid.

GRAZIELLA

Everyday life in Italy is organized around families; a global pandemic could hardly change this fact. Solidarity thus involves not only the usual lot of young adult "activists", but also youngsters, grandparents, cousins and more. Graziella, me and my husband's "nonna," lives near us in the Friuli Venezia-Giulia region. As an 86-year-old, she belongs to one of the most at-risk groups for COVID-19. Yet she maintains a sensibility of solidarity and optimism.

> With the virus – according to me – the people have changed for the better. When this thing goes away, the people will be changed. It's not a small thing that's happening. It's truly scary, this disease. And it's global; it's not only in Italy. That's what gives me fear. Will we come out of this period with this virus? I don't know. Let's hope for the best. We all have to have courage. All of us, Americans, English, we all have to have courage. All of us. Things will be different now. It will be another life.

IRENE

Irene is a university student and an organizer of the Lena-Modotti Brigade in Milan, one of largest and most expensive cities in Italy, and one of the cities most severely impacted by Covid-19 in the world. Before the pandemic, Irene had two jobs but has since lost both. Lena-Modotti is one of ten such solidarity brigades throughout Milan. Each is responsible for several sections or "zones" of the city. Lena-Modotti operates out of the Lambretta squat, where Irene lives with her compatriots. Like Ritmo Lento, Lambretta, is associated with the Arci Network, a nationwide web of youth centers. Lena-Modotti provides the same core services as Don't Panic! including collecting and organizing groceries, medicine and supplies for vulnerable individuals and families confined to their homes.

> It is a very powerful project that involves many people. We are over 200 volunteers, from students to workers,

but especially university students. Each zone of Milan has its own brigade and each has its own name and organization. We work in Zones 2 and 3. But each one has a particular style, also for the communication especially. It is a diverse set of political perspectives, groups that are usually always in competition, but now are working together. The Lena-Modotti Brigade is one of the most organized because of Lambretta. We communicate with each other, teach and inform each other about what needs to be done.

How do you feel when you do this work?
I feel very happy and very politically active and present in the city during this emergency. Every day, every week, it grows bigger. At first, we were bringing grocery shopping to people who cannot go out or because they are at risk or for other difficulties, but we are collecting food for people who are suffering because of the economic crisis.

We created an emergency phone line with 80 operators to talk with people who are in the worst situations. The people that telephone us are often from Sri Lanka and the Philippines and now Arabic people are also beginning to contact us for Ramadan. Every day we get on the phone and explain to the people that contact us about our project and how the collection of food is organized. They request food like rice, juices, something energetic, nutritious food, flour, couscous, and vegetables. And we put in these packages of food pasta, tomato sauce, tuna, biscuits, and also personal health products like toothbrushes and toilet paper.

The work of an operator is very stressful. Every day, we receive approximately 200 or 300 calls. We are so many people, but it is a difficult job because so many people call. Every time you must repeat the same things, while also figuring out the situation of the person. Usually they are women, and they don't know Italian very well, so it is even difficult to communicate. We had an overwhelming number of requests at the beginning. In fact, we had to select the people to help first depending on their economic situation. We had to prioritize people with children, old folks, or based on the number of people in the house. They are difficult decisions.

Do you think this project will persist after the immediate crisis?
Yes, this project will continue in the long term. We don't know exactly for how long, because no one knows the future. Until June surely. But we want to maintain this project if we can because every day there is a lot of work to do. And everything is voluntary, no payments, no earnings. So it is a problem for us, because every one of us is a student, a worker, or a person who is precarious [*precario*]. But the perspective will go on. We are thinking to make an association, a collaboration pact [*patto di collaborationze*] with the municipality of Milan, basically to have a legal place to do these things for other emergencies.

How should things change?
The experience of the brigades must be a turning point, an impetus for reflection by everyone about all of the

struggles we've fought until now. Because the state took everything from us [over the years], and it has been totally absent during this moment of emergency. Only the work of solidarity has helped the poorest people. The lowest classes are the ones who are paying for what the government hasn't been able to do. The ones who do this work are solidarity people [*persone solidale*] like us who understood the situation and entered the field to help – even though it is risking our lives.

The level of active solidarity that bloomed between people exceeded my highest expectation. I would have never expected this nor the degree to which we are now recognized by the community. For example, the Filipino community recognizes us as an important actor to interface with because we are present and we really can help. It's very important that we've arrived to help these minorities during this period when people are forced to be home. The fact we have created a web of solidarity that is able to reach the most vulnerable and precarious during this crisis – it's a great achievement.

With the recent easing of lockdown measures, Italians are re-emerging from their homes to a society with profoundly changed attitudes and expectations. Both Don't Panic and the Lena-Modotti Brigade are well on their way to securing collaboration pacts with their respective municipalities, agreements that will no doubt seed new horizontal civic projects in response to Covid-19 and beyond.

CHAPTER TEN

Solidarity Networks in Greece

EP and TP

We were looking for guns/ we knew/ all die/ but there exist deaths that burden/ because they choose the way./ And we decided/ death to death/ because we loved life a lot. (Katerina Gogou, *Three Clicks Left*, 1978, 13)[1]

February 25, 2020, emergency legislation is rushed in. February 26, the Greek health ministry confirms the first case of Covid-19. Then, three phases. The first, February 27–March 22, when Greek politicians hedge. They individualize responsibility and declare Covid-19 an "invisible enemy" and the second front in the current war, the "asymmetrical threat" of immigration. The second phase, March 23–May 3, a curfew is in effect throughout Greece, monitored by police. In the absence of any prevention or treatment, the state resorts to physical-distancing measures and movement restrictions. Testing is reserved for those at risk of developing severe disease and vulnerable populations – limited really to critical or hospitalized cases. Little to no protective provisions for healthcare workers, much less anyone else who does not work remotely. No protection for prisoners or immigration detainees. The third phase, May 4–, a gradual rollback of the lockdown is attempted, a new normal for flexible work with reductions in work time and pay.

We refrain from talking of failure or negligence but, rather, see behind the Covid-19 and health system burdens. The Greek state has distributed these burdens unevenly in order to conciliate opposing interests and balance them out in time – short term for constituents, medium term for the electoral cycle, and long term for capital accumulation. Covid-19 is not only a matter of virulence and infectivity, but a result of global industrial agriculture with unchecked pathogens. Greece has experienced a decrease in life expectancy and underdeveloped primary health-care even before austerity and cuts (2010–20), in the interests of the wealthy and to placate the EU. This current crisis creates an even greater crisis as those forced to work matter the most; those forcibly unemployed matter the least; and the invisible, sometimes objects of work, do not matter at all. Self-organized solidarity – including but not limited to mobilizations – takes place in all spheres such as workplaces, hospitals, prisons, immigration detention centers, and others.

We interviewed a diverse group of people, all involved in efforts to provide both material support and counter-information, asking them what, why and to whom they provided support and information, how they related the two, what was new (or not), and about the future.

SOCIAL HEALTH CLINICS SOLIDARITY NETWORK[2]

The whole world is in lockdown. Everybody feels a pervading sentiment of fear. Afraid for their lives and for imminent punishment in case of noncompliance to state orders. In this context, we continued efforts with social health clinics created years ago in the aftermath of the financial crisis, creating a solidarity network. Social health clinics are self-organized, bottom-up health clinics operating through horizontal decision making processes, like open general assemblies. Our most important goal is to deploy and project another understanding of health and illness that doesn't distinguish doctors, knowledge holders, and patients who must accept whatever the specialist says. We aim to establish horizontal relationships between care givers and care takers, creating conditions for care takers to become care givers, contributing to the social health clinics' "solidarity chain." We want people to realize that health care is everyone's inalienable right and cannot be commercialized.

During the pandemic's spread, we decided to create a solidarity network connecting efforts in four social health clinics in Athens, one in Thessaloniki and one in Volos. This network expands continuously, connecting existing members with members of recovering addicts and others supporting our aims. Meeting people's needs for food and pharmaceuticals, the network creates online psychological support for people experiencing difficulties in these special circumstances, in housing deprivation or suffering mental illnesses. We are thinking of creating a support network for mothers with young children, responding to their requests.

We are already connected to various counter-information efforts and intend to expand them, creating a special counter-information sub-group. During the coronavirus crisis, government propaganda aims to brainwash people. It's very important to communicate among ourselves, to know what exactly is happening, and why it is happening.

We support people already receiving health care services from clinics, realizing that many can't meet their nutritional needs. We support a wide range of people, receiving calls for help from everywhere. From institutions, like public nursing homes, institutions for people with special needs, but also random people. We don't forget the vulnerable; homeless, addicts, refugees abandoned to their fate.

There are 20,000 people living in Moria camp (Lesvos) meant for 3,000 people. They live under awful conditions, accessing running water only three times per day, with inadequate nutrition and children playing around garbage. The virus reaches some camps, some are quarantined, but the problem remains unsolved. We stand in solidarity with refugees. We can't reach quarantined camps, but we support migrants without papers in Petrou Ralli detention center, providing greatly needed personal hygiene items. We support refugees in the few remaining refugee squats after the government, post-election, "cleaned" Exarchia.

We don't do philanthropy. This network doesn't only provide material support. It has an essential role in strengthening social ties weakened due to social distancing; in strengthening communication; in strengthening our decision to stand up for everybody; uniting our power; preparing for tomorrow; not succumbing to the fear that the ones 'above' cultivate. This pandemic is a turning point. We are ready for tomorrow. The movement in Greece has very good reflexes. People responded very quickly through various efforts, showing great persistence in resistance, filling us with optimism. (K.M. and V.K., members of the social health clinic of Patision, Athens)

KRAH, CHANIA, COMMUNITY RADIO, CRETE[3]

The Chania Community Radio[4] is self-identified as a horizontal, self-organized, noncommercial, anti-racist and anti-sexist project with a clear political aim to negotiate the opening of a social spectrum for voices less heard.

During the pandemic, our goal "to give voice to those who don't have one" became critical. Although KRaH as a collective has not offered material solidarity, its members have done so in many different ways. Our program speaks to and about those either not represented by mainstream TV and radio channels or who have seen their viewpoints critically altered and heavily manipulated.

KRaH Radio addresses those who want to know what is happening in an unmediated way and to hear or play something new, leaving a different musical, political and aesthetic mark.

As the public sphere was occupied by the dominant discourse, during the pandemic we felt utterly uncomfortable. After discussing the pandemic's political and financial impact, the "reaction of the state" (oppression) but also watching the panic spread, we realized that a calm, grounded voice to communicate a broader understanding of the situation was essential.

This motivated us to support and nurture relations among the oppressed, setting the ground for solidarity. In order to give voice to the unheard, to strengthen collectives and self-organized structures that had just started to flourish, we embarked on:

- A daily counter-information newscast, consisting of announcements of the antagonistic movement, lived experiences about confinement, fear and domination during the Covid-19 period; and news about workers and the oppressed, immigrants and incarcerated people.
- A weekend newscast with "personal voices" publicized in social media, blogs and webpages.
- Our health newscast, without dramatic music or imperatives – simple rules like the WHO suggests, useful phone lines and web platforms providing free psychological support.
- Web shows and discussions related to coronavirus and its impact.
- Promotion of local collectives providing material solidarity.
- Denouncements of pandemic police arbitrariness and abuse of power against civilians and state negligence.
- Tributes to lost militants who left an important legacy (Periklis Korovesis, Helin Bölek, İbrahim Gökçek, Mustafa Koçak, Manolis Glezos).

We believe that material support is based on trust built when you listen and you are respectfully heard, when both individual and collective opinions are heard. In a state of emergency, it is important to make our voices strong and offer a framework to help as many voices as possible to be heard. Counter-information connects people and the radio is a vivid means to convey society's nerve. Building on this, we come first to know each other and, furthermore, to provide material support. We built a non-antagonistic public sphere "sans spectacle."

Confinement has made mutual support essential and in KRaH we communicate daily with one another, organize the daily newscast and discuss personal and general difficulties as well as lived experiences. In addition, our weekly assembly meeting gives us the opportunity to discuss political issues and seek common ground. While all this existed previously, in the Covid-19 era it became a daily routine for participants in our assembly and radio broadcasts.

During this intense time, we have created dynamic communication not only within our group but also with the people we address, a regular communication with collectives, unions and individuals. It is our wish that this will continue after the crisis, fulfilling KRaH's initial goal – to make marginalized voices heard: in a space of active and honest dialogue among people and collectives where shared opinions and perspectives develop daily inside the movement both in difficult times and times of a contrived and catastrophic "normality."

We have not reached our dream. In fact, we are very far from it. And that is not due to our low expectations or our inability to succeed – though we are realists regarding our prospects and our limited resources – but mostly because our dreams have no limits. We have made steps that seemed very difficult to some of us. Currently, the greatest difficulties are behind us. As long as our group grows bigger, our effort broader, and the quietest of the voices get heard, this effort and its necessity will embrace our society. (KRaH, Chania Community Radio assembly)

SOLIDARITY FUND FOR IMPRISONED AND PERSECUTED MILITANTS[5]

The Solidarity Fund for Imprisoned and Persecuted Militants is a political structure established in 2010 under conditions of harsh capitalist restructuring, through the vehicle of "economic crisis," and a blooming radical movement, remembering social revolts of December 2008. Under those circumstances, repression intensified, resulting in ever-increasing numbers of political prisoners. Our aim is to provide regular, consistent support to those persecuted or imprisoned for participating in social and class struggles, and for subversive action in the revolutionary struggle, including struggles in prisons. We have always stood with persecuted militants, covering part of their court expenses and bail. We consider important political and practical support to migrants systematically made illegal and imprisoned in concentration camps by the state.

We try to consistently deal with every difficulty that we encounter, based on comradeship and solidarity.

We intervene politically via events, book presentations, publications, and translations of books and texts written by imprisoned comrades. For many years we have published the quarterly *Tearing Down Bastille*, which included texts by imprisoned comrades. We have participated in word and actions in struggles of imprisoned comrades against vindictive penalties, solitary confinement, transfer and torture. We support calls to be present at court and political trials, with our words or physical presence, because for us, it is an urgent need not to leave them alone against the civil state.

Our basic aim is to ensure decent living conditions for imprisoned comrades by political action, taking material solidarity a step beyond close family, friendly and comrade relationships. We provide practical solidarity, build communication bridges and common struggles between prisoners and those outside. We achieve this by organizing events with current and former imprisoned comrades, publishing print material, and various social actions of solidarity and support. Our imprisoned comrades are a vital part of the broader antagonistic movement. Solidarity isn't only material, but also ethical and political.

In the current pandemic and restrictive measures imposed by the state, we face an unprecedented situation domestically and globally. In the imposed curfew, we were forced to suspend all our planned public actions, extremely difficult not only because we couldn't ensure material support, but also because we couldn't abandon those facing repressive mechanisms and dangerous conditions risking their health. Overcrowding of Greek prisons, inadequate or non-existent medical care, few personal protective measures, continued confinement even for the most vulnerable – all created conditions for significantly high mortality rates, which may amount to the death penalty for many prisoners.

Consequently, a series of prison mobilizations escalated to the women's prison in Thiva in response to a prisoner's death and spread throughout other prisons. Prisoners abstained from work and meals and refused to enter cells. The key demands were decongestion of prisons and implementation of basic protection measures. Meanwhile, communication with the outside was blocked by suspending visits from relatives and lawyers. Retaliatory measures continued against outbreaks of protest, culminating in cases of abductions and transfers of comrades, of militants.

After years of continuous persecutions and imprisonments, the Solidarity Fund is more topical and necessary than ever. We stand against the crime of incarceration that reproduces class inequalities, fear and submission. Following Covid-19 the Solidarity Fund faces a serious problem concerning the viability of financially supporting imprisoned militants. We need financial support from the global movement. We won't work less than before, because solidarity can't be put in quarantine. We have a long way to go, but the slogan "no one left alone in the hands of the state" is more crucial and tangible than ever. Factual solidarity will again be our weapon. (E.L., member of the Solidarity Fund for Imprisoned and Persecuted Militants)

CLASS COUNTER ATTACK (ANARCHIST AND COMMUNIST GROUP)[6]

As of April 2020, Greece's public health system isn't severely affected by the spread of coronavirus. Rather it's suffering financially due to the general lockdown and production freeze, on top of a decade of deep impoverishment and increased anti-labor, anti-popular policies in the aftermath of the 2010 default. The neoliberal onslaught, complying with the EU's orders, literally destroyed the public health system. While EUR 44 bn has been spent on the army (2009–19), public health care expenditure decreased 42 percent. These aren't just statistics, but capitalism's core logic.

So, the organized movement must act in two reciprocal directions by active resistance, breaking the state's monopoly of violence, and developing social and class solidarity structures. Class Counter Attack's structure organizes solidarity actions supporting people severely affected by the crisis (refugees, immigrants, elders in nursing homes, families in need) and politically supporting Turkish and Kurdish political refugees oppressed by the Greek state, elder militants of the anti-fascist and anti-imperialist guerilla struggle (1941–49), the Solidarity Fund for Imprisoned and Persecuted Militants and refugee squat Notara 26.

Within the suffocating ambience of quarantine, our group chose to remain politically active, exploring every possibility for public action. Beyond social and class solidarity actions, we participate in solidarity actions for public health care system workers, labor unions, refugees in concentration camps, imprisoned comrades in suffocating conditions, and organize mobilizations and uprisings. Similarly, our counter-information actions support workers, unemployed, poor people, excluded and oppressed people, those deprived of a voice and basic rights, those who "do not have a mouth and must scream." Created in 2014, we have experience in solidarity actions from the 2015–16 "refugee crisis" when we created solidarity structures to materially support refugees and immigrants. For us, solidarity is neither a charity nor a humanitarian organization.

Counter-information isn't simple but breaking the state's monopoly on discourse is a fundamental duty – to analyze what's happening now and what will happen in the upcoming economic crash and new attacks on labor and people, shifting the crisis to poor people. This analysis is not for academia or record keeping, but to guide a political strategy that aims to rupture the world of capital, state, and social revolution. It's a difficult and steep route, back and forth, and many in-between stops. Conflicts with state and capital, developing structures of social and class solidarity, mutual aid, theory, analysis and counter-information can't be separated. They should form a coherent and dialectical whole.

Despite 10 years' experience of continuous capitalist crisis, as a circumstantial turning point this pandemic crisis is yet to be explored. We will take qualitative and organizational steps to fulfill new duties. Nothing is easy, but also nothing is impossible. A field of new possibilities are opening and we must be ready to turn people's inevitable discontent in a revolutionary and progressive direction (not conservatism, fascism and social democracy, as with the previous cycle of struggles following the Greek state's default in 2010). The pandemic has definitely created a difficult and suffocating situation. We should be careful in our moves because, besides state oppression, lost human lives won't come back. But we shall never forget: hope is always in the streets ... (P.G, member of Class Counter Attack)

NOTES

1. K. Gogou, "Three Clicks Left, 13". In *Let's See What You Are Going to Do Now, Poems 1978–2002*. 2012. Athens: Kastaniotis, p. 26.
2. https://iatreioapa.blogspot.com/; email: iatreioapa@gmail.com.
3. https://kpaxradio.live/; email: kpaxradio@gmail.com.
4. Both our name (the initials in Greek echo the "Crash of 29" or any other major economic disaster) and our slogan "KRaH in the dominant frequencies" reflect this.
5. www.tameio.org/; www.firefund.net/imprisonedsoli; email: tameio@espiv.net.
6. https://taksiki-antepithesi.espivblogs.net/; email: taksiki-antepithesi@espiv.net.

CHAPTER ELEVEN

Viral Solidarity: Experiences from the UK

Neil Howard

In the UK, the corona crisis is having a range of devastating impacts which are playing out along lines traced by existing inequalities. Millions have lost their jobs, large numbers are unable to pay their rent, and some of the poorest and most marginalized are having to risk their health by continuing to work so as not to starve. On top of this, domestic violence has increased, some of the sick are unable to be treated, and of course many are dying.

Yet within the suffering and dislocation, beautiful things have emerged. There has been a nationwide eruption of localized mutual aid groups connecting via digital platforms such as Facebook to ensure provision of basic needs for those unable to secure them. These groups are organized by residential locality so that previously disconnected dwellings are becoming neighborhoods in the process of providing each other with support. One recent survey found that more than 80 percent of people aged over 70 had been offered such support to get through this period.[1]

Similarly, over a million people have volunteered to help the National Health Service (NHS), which is as close to a state religion as exists in the UK. Volunteers have stepped forward to perform previously uncelebrated tasks such as cleaning and waste disposal, and a number of "good news stories" have circulated documenting how many people from high status professions have volunteered for humble jobs so as to be useful at this time.

Progressive political organizing is receiving a significant boost, too. Activists, campaigning organizations and left-leaning politicians all recognize that this crisis is an unparalleled opportunity, both to build a more caring society and to usher in the much-needed green transition to a post-carbon economy. More and more people are aware that the former status quo left too many vulnerable and uncared for and therefore want change. This is seeing a huge rise in calls for policies such as Unconditional Basic Income (UBI), for increased funding of public services, and even for bold measures to tackle climate collapse. Encouragingly, movements such as Green New Deal UK are building cross-sectional coalitions with those engaged in other struggles (like labor unions) towards a more fundamental reconfiguration of the UK's social settlement.

A vital thread linking all of the above is the return of shared human needs to the foreground of public and political consciousness. In particular, needs for care, community, meaning and hope appear to be back on the collective radar. In pre-crisis times, much of what went by the name of "work" neither cared for anything nor gave anyone a sense of meaning, while a deep sense of community was difficult for many to experience in the midst of the alienation and speed of life on the capitalist treadmill. Each of these facts combined to make life feel hopeless for millions, with the possibility of things being different foreclosed in the seeming inevitability of neoliberal life.

Right now, in the midst of crisis, all of this is changing for large numbers of people. For those whose work is usually meaningless, slowdown and crisis are offering an opportunity not only to reflect on how dissatisfying "ordinary" life is but to take actions which care for others and therefore convey a sense of meaning. In turn, many people are discovering a sense of community in serving those they may not previously have been connected to. Combined, these facts prefigure a different way of organizing our society and that is seeing the return of tentative but very tangible hope – and on a previously unimaginable scale.

The four interviewees whose voices comprise the majority of this chapter all speak to the return of hope and to the centrality of care in this return. Although all are from very different backgrounds (and indeed countries), they are united in using their individual energies in the service of wider collectives. Their contributions range in size and in scale, with two dedicated to organizing in their localities, one contributing to nationwide campaigns, and a fourth organizing transnationally. I am connected to each of them in different ways and inspired by them all. We begin with Margaret Howard, my mum.[2]

MARGARET HOWARD, LOCAL LABOUR COUN-CILLOR, SAMARITAN AND RETIRED TEACHER

I quickly realized that coronavirus was going to leave a lot of people in a very vulnerable position. So, I started a Facebook support group to bring people together and link those who needed help with those who could offer it. Very quickly the group had offers and I created a googledoc matching the names to the roads. From that I made files for several of the busiest roads so we all knew who to ask. By the evening of the first day we decided to make a leaflet [and] pretty soon the whole of our neighbourhood and half of the next were leafleted, which was about 7000 households. The outpouring of love from everyone and the need to help was extraordinary.

During all this I heard that Community House was to be closed. This was a social hub which also acted as a foodbank for those who fell outside the system. I knew that closing it would be a disaster, so with several friends looked for alternative accommodation and funds. There are now ten people involved and a temporary foodbank which is fully operational in a local church – all within a week. It's amazing.

I'm not really sure what motivated me to do this, now that you ask, as it has all happened so fast! I remember that I just wanted to make sure vulnerable people weren't left worrying about their future as this disease was known to be worse for the elderly and people with health issues. Thinking about people being stuck indoors on their own, possibly without family, and not knowing how they could get their shopping or prescriptions, made me question what I could do to help. I knew that the situation needed someone who could help with the coordination so I decided to fill that role, given that my own age and health means that I have to isolate and cannot do other things.

It has been very tiring because it has been relentless, but underneath that it has made me feel useful, like I am contributing something to the wellbeing of others. So that's a good feeling, without which I imagine it would be easy to lose hope and get depressed.

N: Although this crisis is causing a lot of pain and suffering, many people seem to be connecting to hope. Has this been your experience?
M: Without doubt this has opened up a whole generation to caring about others. The need to support neighbours and the vulnerable. The "me me me" emphasis has been replaced with we and us. It's very heart-warming. Suddenly the most important thing is how we support each other. Empathy for doctors, nurses, care workers, waste disposal workers, it has all risen, as has the realization that money isn't everything.

I hope that things have changed forever. I hope more people appreciate that the government has been failing us and now see the people and services that matter. Think of the NHS, of the fire service, police, railways, buses, education, which should be financially rewarded over the banks, corporations and insurance companies that shouldn't. I hope the government will have the courage to refuse to financially help the companies that trade offshore and don't pay taxes. If not now, then when?

The response from the public has been phenomenal and proves that giving people enough time and space leaves them room to think of others. They are desperate to reach out and help others. It's a joy to behold and gives me hope that it has opened people's eyes to what is important. The thought that it won't is unbearable to contemplate.

CATHERINE HEINEMEYER, STORYTELLER, DRAMA PRACTITIONER, ACADEMIC

I research and teach the role of storytelling in education, mental health and in relation to the ecological crisis. I've also been involved with Extinction Rebellion (XR) over the past two years. I'd been an activist in my teens and early twenties, but subsequently more or less lost hope that a mass movement for a just transition would form in time to make a meaningful difference. That was particularly bitter as I was raising my own children then. But by demanding what is necessary rather than what seems possible, XR and the school strike movement have reawakened hope – in me and in many others.

I have at least three people living inside my head right now: an anxious extrovert who finds lockdown a tremendous strain and can't wait for it to end, a commonsensical roll-your-sleeves-up type getting involved in local initiatives and trying to support my neighbours, and a hopeful revolutionary who sees the real possibility that this enforced pause is our best chance to reset our economy and politics – to turn the tanker round towards a liveable future.

Lots of things that we were told were impossible happened within days when a genuine threat was perceived: people's wellbeing has been put above economic growth, homelessness was essentially ended overnight in the UK, most of the airplanes stopped flying and the cars stopped driving. This is unprecedented.

Since this all started, I've been involved in national online conversations through XR to make sure that the post-Covid rebuild brings us to a different kind of economy and politics. There is a huge, understandable desire in society to get back to "normal," and this will be shouted particularly loudly by those whose interests were served by that version of normality, even if it was really a crisis and an emergency.

To build a genuinely mass movement, I'm convinced that we need to tell another story, one of the just and sustainable society that is still, to some extent, possible. We also need to align the stories we tell as much as possible, so that different communities and constituencies hear the same hopeful narratives. So, I have been helping to facilitate a regular online discussion of green NGOs, and also working with some wonderful collaborators on a short animated film which will encapsulate some of these ideas in an accessible, shareable, metaphorical way – a story, in other words.

N: Amen! And what are you experiencing in your life during the crisis that makes you believe a new story of solidarity could take hold?
C: Well there's lots of inspiring local action happening, some of which I'm connected to. For example, when tonnes of overwintered potatoes couldn't be harvested a few weeks ago, people I know at Abundance York organized forty volunteers to go and harvest them for distribution to food banks.

Also, when my youth theatre group could no longer meet, a fellow drama practitioner at York Theatre Royal connected me with Shpresa, an organization supporting refugee young people in London. I now tell stories to a sparky little girl twice a week on videocall – we have a brilliant time writing stories together too – to help her keep up her English and let her imagination fly, and to try and give her mum a boost as well. I sincerely hope Shpresa is typical of other groups supporting vulnerable people in isolation – within a few weeks it has transformed all its services to keep young asylum seekers and refugees connected, learning, safe and active during this really challenging time. As you and I have discussed now many times, this is all about care and hope!

JACEY HEARN, STUDENT, DISABILITY SUPPORT WORKER, ANTI-FASCIST

My first reaction to the news of coronavirus was to dismiss it. That changed quickly and I was overcome with the question: "What the hell are we going to do?" My work and activism exposed me to information about how big this was going to be, so I started looking for what to do. I have asthma and knew that I wouldn't be able to help people in person, so I joined the nascent Mutual Aid group in my town and have been crazily busy with it ever since.

It's a city-wide network, now broken down into neighbourhoods and streets, coordinating the mutual provision of support, with specific attention to groups who are often marginalized by state offerings. It has grown so rapidly and has thousands of people engaged in doing all sorts of things. I have been very involved in setting up the platform, forming the groups, doing the spreadsheets – very much the in-the-background stuff that often gets forgotten but is also essential.

N: It sounds like you're very connected to a sense of responsibility ...
J: I always say, "If not now then, when?" and "If not us, then who?" and I feel both of these questions very strongly at this time, especially as a time of crisis is also a time of opportunity ... My background is in anarchist politics and although I'm loving seeing the care and self-organization that is flourishing now, I'm constantly irked that we weren't able to create the container for this to develop before. Like, how come we couldn't catalyse people's care at this scale without a pandemic?

N: Yes, totally. And, of course, this also begs the question, "How do we keep this stuff going?"
J: Absolutely. That question is constantly in my head and in our movement, and the Mutual Aid Network is having weekly meetings about it. These are super useful and for some have been transformative. We know we want to keep the best of this going, we know we need to find our space, and we know we have to work out how to engage the state without being co-opted.

My absolute dream is that everyone will finally understand that they can act autonomously, do good when they do so, and keep doing it. I dream that we will all see that we have power in and of ourselves and that we have power in community, which is better and more beautiful than everyday capitalist life. In reality, I know this isn't how it will play out. So, I guess my more grounded hope is that this experience is planting millions of seeds that will germinate in an awareness and desire to struggle towards the better world that we have now experienced and want to keep.

VIBHOR MATHUR, PH.D STUDENT, ACTIVIST

Pre-Covid life for me was reasonably busy – I'm a Ph.D student in the UK, run an education and community mobilization NGO called Spinning Wheel Leadership Foundation in India, and am engaged in environmental and political activism in both countries. Right now, while my Ph.D work continues (roughly) uninterrupted, my NGO work has shifted massively and, in many ways, increased. Likewise, my activism.

On top of the usual, I'm involved in three additional projects. The first is trying to co-facilitate a global campaign for emergency basic income. The economic hardships that people are suffering are unimaginable, and definitely beyond the remit of the narrow "recovery" policies that governments are planning. What this involves is running www.emergencybasicincome.com as a platform to collate resources, people, campaigns, ideas and networks of basic income campaigns and campaigners across the world.

Second, I'm involved with the UK network of basic income activists. This is an inspiring and motivated group of experts, organizers, academics and citizens who are spearheading different efforts to try and push the government towards a basic income here.

Finally, I'm conducting a research project in Muslim neighbourhoods in Jaipur, India. This aims to challenge the rampant and misinformed Islamophobia around the spread of Covid-19 in India.

N: These are all very cool initiatives. Can you say more about the "why" behind your engagement?

V: It's quite difficult for me to pin down why I do what I do. The short, uncritical answer is that it makes me feel happy, fulfilled and purpose-driven. The longer answer is that when I first began becoming aware of structural inequality, it felt "wrong" to not do what I could to battle it. I'm aware that so much of my life is a product of historical and structural privileges that I continue to enjoy. That awareness puts a fire in my belly.

N: And what's the feeling as you do what you do?

V: In a strange way, it's empowering to be fighting against structures and institutions that seem too strong to collapse. Equally, it's empowering to feel the optimism that one day the world could be better. That hope is a fuel which is both free and unending and is therefore a continuous source of motivation. The obvious problem with that is that it is mostly internal, reinforced only by small victories and the networks I can create. There are days when I'm exhausted, when I read one piece of news and just collapse.

N: I hear that, a balance between hope and overwhelm ...

V: Exactly. And, you know, adjusting and getting to grips with lockdown has made a lot of people question what they considered to be "normal," "valuable" or "productive." Equally, people are having to imagine and rely on social, filial and community networks to tide them through. I have also seen a much higher degree of concern for those most vulnerable either to the virus or its socio-economic fallouts. In trying to strike the balance between supporting governments in their efforts to stop the virus and questioning whether they are doing enough, people are being more active as citizens than when the humdrum of daily life drowned out non-work-related concerns. All of these hopeful things encourage me that people have taken this time to pause, rethink and (hopefully) imagine a better future.

N: Do you think we will be able to sustain these positive changes?

V: This is something I wrestle with every day, and honestly, I don't know. On the one hand, I want to be optimistic and think that what and who people value will shift. We will recognize what jobs matter more. We will cherish ourselves, our families, our wellbeing, our support networks. We will be more active as citizens. But the devil on the other shoulder is more pessimistic. The fabric of our "lifestyles" is built by the capitalist-democratic project to be centred around output. This means that priorities, systems and our lives are shaped by those who have an interest in returning us to the previous status quo. This worries me because our politicians seem to believe that an industry-led recovery of the economy is the way to go. My hope is that at an individual level we can maintain the aforementioned changes, and across societies make this strong enough to push for major reforms to what we once considered "normal."

Thank you for this, Neil. It has been an emotional churn to try and answer these questions, but one that I've really enjoyed. This is probably the first time since the pandemic started that I've been able to stop and reflect on what's happening inside my heart and mind.

If you want to know more about or be involved with any of the initiatives mentioned in this chapter, please search online – all have websites full of information.

NOTES

1. See the UK Office of National Statistics: www.ons.gov.uk/peoplepopulationandcommunity/healthandsocialcare/healthandwellbeing/bulletins/coronavirusandthesocialimpactsongreatbritain/9april2020#main-points (accessed April 26, 2020).
2. All four participants gave their fully informed consent for me to interview them and reproduce their words in this chapter. One interviewee, Jacey, requested that they be anonymized, which they have, through that pseudonym.

PART V

Turtle Island (North America)

CHAPTER TWELVE

Turtle Island

carla bergman and magalí rabasa
with Ariella Patchen and Seyma Özdemir

> All that you touch
> You Change.
> All that you Change,
> Changes you.
> The only lasting truth
> is Change.
>
> (Octavia Butler)

Turtle Island is the name many Indigenous peoples give to the landmass known as North America. So, we begin this chapter with a question: why think about Turtle Island and not individual countries like the other chapters in this collection? At the core, it is a recognition of ongoing colonialism, and ongoing cross-border resistance throughout Turtle Island. We also want to intentionally decenter the settler-colonial state, and in particular the US.

The ongoing economic and political fallout will undoubtedly be long-lasting, demanding that we connect and build relations of support beyond our usual networks and collective capacities, across all kinds of borders. The fallout and ensuing tragedies will not be equally distributed across North America. We must think and act beyond border imperialism. While the fascist doctrine of "America First" is making the US the new center of the pandemic, we want to listen to the voices of those most impacted by the effects of the pandemic within and beyond the US borders. We also want to listen to those communities that are actively constructing autonomous practices of mutual aid. While the official responses to the pandemic, from above, actively work to mark the differences between countries, reinforcing and indeed even closing borders, the view from below tells a different story, which is a story of solidarity and mutual aid, a story of resonances and connections that reach across borders and across territories.

Given the quick timeline of this project, we opted to work with folks in spaces where trust was already established. As such, the interviews and stories here, while inspiring and powerful, are not included because we think they're the most important ones to amplify. We recognize that there are countless actions happening every day, and many in subtle and quiet ways, and we give our deepest gratitude to everyone being there for each other during the pandemic.

All of the interviews in this chapter happened in April 2020. We interviewed folks who are close friends, or friends of friends, crossing over the borders. After interviewing Indigenous folks from various communities, a thread emerged that spoke to a decolonial solidarity amid the ongoing colonialism throughout Turtle Island, one that predates anarchist versions of mutual aid. These different yet equally inspiring lifeways can show us all that we can collectively embrace deepening solidarity in our lives as we move through this time and towards a more grounded future.

The majority of the interviews were conducted and edited by us, but we've also included three sections by collaborators, Ariella Patchen, Dani Burlison and Seyma Özdemir. As we think beyond nation-state logics, we've chosen to organize the interviews in clusters around six interconnected themes:

- Indigenous organizing across Turtle Island
- Organizing in immigrant communities
- Prisoner solidarity
- Online mutual aid networks
- Mutual aid among people who are unhoused and precariously housed
- Autonomous health organizing.

The situation we are facing is new terrain, requiring us to show up in new and unforeseen ways for and with each other. It's been powerful to see folks adapt and be there for each other all over the world. The kinds of solidarity and mutual aid that have emerged are truly extraordinary and awe-inspiring, and outweigh all the shitty news we hear every day. For us, it is the light in these very dark times. At its core, solidarity means listening; it's an action, it's active. And when we spoke with folks for this book, that's what rang through – a deep commitment to listening to each other as they traverse these unknown and turbulent paths to provide support and care for each other. Through a collective commitment to a profound responsibility for each other starting in our neighborhoods, we have seen that there are many hopeful cracks that are allowing infinite possibilities to emerge, and with which we can imagine and enact a better world together, post-Covid-19. Maybe even undoing colonialism once and for all.

NO ONE WAS UNSHELTERED BEFORE 1492

Klee Benally (Diné/Navajo) is a volunteer with Táala Hooghan Infoshop and Kinlani/Flagstaff Mutual Aid, and a writer, musician and filmmaker. "This is a humanitarian crisis, and so all people without shelter in this pandemic should be considered refugees."

Describe your activities since the beginning of the outbreak of Covid-19.

On March 14th, inspired by the amazing mutual aid mobilizations throughout Turtle Island, I contacted a local street medic crew to see about interest in initiating a localized project. That was the spark we needed. The framework for mutual aid groups was already established, we just needed a model to draw and build from. It happened organically as an extension of work we had been doing out of Táala Hooghan Infoshop since 2007.

We built a Facebook group and Google form, and borrowed from the DC Mutual Aid framework of establishing a Hub (to coordinate volunteers and requests), a supply site (Táala Hooghan infoshop), and delivery (from the volunteer forms). We scoured the web for the best protocols, compiling enough info and resources to spring into action. Since then Kinlani (Flagstaff)

Mutual Aid has grown, doing daily support throughout the region.

As politicians in the so-called "U.S." urged people to stock-up on 2 weeks of supplies, my relative Ethel Branch saw the looming crisis. For the Diné and Hopi reservations, with a population base of about 200,000 people, there are only 13 grocery stores. And as greedy hoarders left shelves empty in the settlements on the periphery of the reservation, she knew there could be a crisis for our elders. She quickly coordinated a GoFundMe for Diné and Hopi elders, gaining an amazing amount of momentum. We connected and I started coordinating out of Táala Hooghan. We mobilized Kinlani Mutual Aid volunteers to gather supplies, deliver food, and sanitize entire trucks. This was right before the tragedy in Chilchinbito on our reservation.

On March 18th, two cases of Covid-19 were confirmed in this incredibly remote Diné community. We now have 1,540 cases on the rez. per capita, if you compare our population to so-called U.S. states, we are the third impacted after New Jersey and New York.

My priorities right now are our elders and unsheltered relatives. Most businesses are shut down in Flagstaff. Most of the resources for unsheltered folks are not available to them except the shelters – where they kick our relatives out at 5 am and treat them worse than most kennels treat animals. The negligence is abhorrent. The Flagstaff politicians had no plan for unsheltered relatives. I've been on the ground at Táala Hooghan every day talking with them and locating resources. That work led me to build emergency wash stations. I made a zine, and now it's being shared across Turtle Island as a simple DIY model for basic hygiene.

Is your work based on ongoing values and principles?
The idea of collective care and support, of ensuring the well-being of all our relations in non-hierarchical voluntary association, and taking direct action has always been something that translated easily for me. That's how I was raised. T'áá hwó' ají t'éego means if it is going to be, it is up to you. No one will do it for you. We also have a Diné philosophy rooted in Ké, or our familial relations, which means that no one would ever be left to fend for themselves, we are all relatives in some way so we have to care for each other. We built these understandings into Táala Hooghan Infoshop from the beginning.

How have you and others adapted to this situation?
It's not so much about adapting as it is about scaling our efforts to meet the critical needs of our people. The crisis around Covid-19 has magnified the existing crises of capitalism and colonialism. It is hardest to address the safety protocols with unsheltered relatives, some of whom may have substance use issues or mental health issues. That's an ongoing process of working with a community that depends in many ways on social proximity for survival. The Navajo Nation also has significant infrastructure challenges: 1/3 of households don't have running water or electricity. Internet access is also limited in many remote areas so the organizing has to be more direct or rely on other channels such as radio.

What's been most surprising and inspiring? What's been challenging?

I'm surprised and inspired every day on how widely the concept of mutual aid has spread. On one hand, there's a level of non-profit and liberal cooptation, but on the other, mutual aid can only really be coopted so much due to the inherent contradictions within settler colonial societies and capitalism. The biggest challenge is how hard our remote communities on the reservation have been hit. Many of these spaces are where our elders live, who do not speak English and continue to be caretakers of our cultural knowledge systems.

Do you think any of these networks will remain beyond the crisis? Beyond the state/charity models?

We're organizing with the vision that these efforts have the power to make capitalism and colonialism irrelevant. We are actively establishing interventions to ensure that these systems don't recuperate. To that end we've established an Indigenous Mutual Aid network (www.indigenousmutualaid.org) to build connections through and beyond this crisis. Since most of the current Indigenous mutual aid organizing is an extension of work that has been ongoing in sacred land and water struggles, for unsheltered relatives, or elder support, we already have a lot of those deep relationships and experiences working together. We want to radically redistribute resources and power but we also don't want to be burdened by leftist political baggage. In many ways that and the threat of non-profit industrial cooptation are perhaps our biggest challenges. That's part of why we're asserting the need for a specific tendency of Indigenous Mutual Aid; we've dealt with white saviors and so much "decolonial" fetishism from radicals. We need them to get out of the way so we can do what we need to do. They have a role, but if we're not organizing on our terms than it's the same charity bullshit we've faced before, no matter how much people say it's "solidarity."

What are your thoughts about creating a more autonomous world that is anti-capitalistic and anti-colonial?
I've grown up in a world of ruins. We have teachings and prophecies of the endings of cycles, but that's always how it's been here. An anti-colonial and anti-capitalist world already exists, but as my father who is a traditional medicine practitioner says, "there aren't two worlds, there is just one world with many paths." Colonial and capitalist paths are linear by design. If that path of greed, domination, exploitation, and competition doesn't accept that it's reached its dead end, then we have to make sure of it.

CHÉNCHENSTWAY IN SOLIDARITY WITH ELDERS

Ta7talíya Michelle Nahanee, S̲k̲wx̲wú7mesh, is a decolonial facilitator and strategist catalyzing social change to transform colonial narratives impacts.

When the pandemic hit, what did you feel called to do?
When we first started feeling the effects of it, all of our workshop bookings were cancelled or postponed. Decolonizing Practices workshops were our main source of income so our livelihood changed dramati-

cally. Every workshop we deliver starts with an Elders'
welcome and blessing. We're proud to give a $400 hon-
orarium for sharing their time and teachings. Many
organizations pay $150 but we intentionally pay more
because we know how many jobs the Elders have to do
each day to survive Vancouver rental costs and living
expenses. And a few of them care for adult children
who are struggling, so the impact multiplies quickly. As
we transitioned to shutting down, we became worried
about our own income, but we were definitely more
worried about the Elders.

We decided to set up a donation option on our website
to try and raise some immediate funds for the Elders.
Within three days we were able to distribute $1200 to
three Coast Salish Elders. As the donations continue to
come in, we forward them, covering transaction fees
as part of our community care. When I first reached
out to share news of the e-transfers, they said "No, no,
that's fine" and "We're fine, don't worry Michelle." They
were more worried for us. Because one of the Elders
had posted about being out $750 that month, I told
her, "You know, it was your post that inspired me to
set this up." There were a few more, "Oh, no, it's fine,
we're fine," and then finally, she said, "Oh, okay." After
I sent the e-transfers, one wrote to me, "I can breathe
now, Michelle." And then what did she do the next
day? She posted about making bannock to bring to the
park to feed Indigenous folks who are experiencing
homelessness.

In our work, we share the teaching of *Chénchenstway*,
it's a Squamish sacred law that means *lifting each other*

up. It's been beautiful to witness the teaching in action and be part of the circle. I'm always talking about the value of Indigenous ways NOW, envisioning ways forward grounded in ways of the lands we occupy. We were able to lift the Elders who have always lifted us. Community has lifted us up with donations and sponsorships for a digital series of our workshops. We've had three philanthropic organizations approach us to sponsor five workshops, which is helping us a lot. So, everything that we share from Squamish values and teachings has come back to us, back to our Elders.

How is Chénchenstway connected to mutual aid and solidarity?
What's interesting is we, *Sk̲wx̲wú7mesh stelmexw*, don't need the words Solidarity or Mutual Aid. *Chénchenstway* is embedded in our lives as a sacred law to live by. Community care and collective wellness is a social norm, so to encourage solidarity or mutual aid would be like encouraging breath. Within our cultural resurgence, we're surfacing these ways, but to be clear, neocolonialism, trauma, and scarcity continue to get in the way. I appreciate the notions of mutual aid and solidarity, and to connect across language and teachings, with the shared meanings and impact of these approaches, keeps me going.

What are your hopes for the future?
I posted a survey on my website asking people *how important it is to decolonize now* and what types of support they wanted from us. I was wondering how relevant our work is and if we should take a break from

the workshops. On the scale of one to ten, nobody rated the importance of decolonization below eight. These are mostly non-Indigenous folks, professionals who are telling us that decolonial approaches are possible and needed. So we'll keep leading that conversation, sharing Indigenous ways for contemporary contexts. I always share that our ways don't just belong in the hunter-gatherer context, they're relevant right now in guiding how we can be better together. More folks are expressing and witnessing beautiful generosity and care – it's contagious, taking us back to the collectivity of our roots.

DECOLONIAL CARE, OR HOW I REALIZED THAT THE MOST RADICAL THING I COULD DO AS A QUEER FEMME OF COLOR WAS TO RADICALLY ACCEPT MY VULNERABILITY, PRACTICE SELF-COMPASSION, AND ACCEPT THE SOLIDARITY BEING OFFERED

Words from an Indigenous educator in Bvlbancha (New Orleans).

As New Orleans began taking precautions to stop the spread of Covid, I was part of the first wave of workers to be laid off. Due to a diagnosis I received in January, I started weekly at-home injections of chemotherapy, and began intensive biologic therapy in late March. The situation was troublesome for me and I was terrified. Not only was I aggressively killing off my entire immune system in the midst of a pandemic, but biweekly, I was going to have to waltz into the hospital that was an epi-center of the virus.

My initial reaction was to postpone treatment, though my doctor explained how that would be more danger-ous. She suggested full self-isolation: no trips to grocery stores or pharmacies. The only time I could go out was to the hospital for treatment.

This was difficult. I was used to jumping into action in response to disasters. I grew up in a rural commu-nity of coastal Louisiana that was frequently battered by increasingly dangerous hurricanes due to climate change. We were frequently neglected by state and federal governments for assistance after these disasters so community mutual aid was an ingrained way of life. There were never discussions about it, you just showed up and did what was needed. I carried this solidarity over to my life in the big city.

With my community quickly becoming the epicenter for the virus, I felt a strong pull to run to the frontlines and help. Except this time I couldn't. Not only was it too dangerous, but it wasn't physically possible. The com-bination of symptoms from illness made functioning daily a struggle. I was exhausted, weak, and experienc-ing physical pain that made standing or walking for extended periods difficult.

Even with all of my anti-colonial, anti-capitalist training, even though I would never look down on someone in my own predicament, I felt like a failure. The long term, intergenerational effects of colonialism had made me sick and capitalism made me feel like it was my own personal failing.

Accepting care is radical.

Over the years, my community has become frustrated with leftist spaces that hyper-focus on theory, single issues, and direct actions while doing little in the way of meaningful community-building and mutual aid. My friend group has spent the last year intentionally creating ways to community-build and set up mutual aid strategies. We envisioned honing these skills in order to better support groups in need when the time for the revolution began. We had no idea it would come so soon, and come in the form of a viral pandemic. I felt lucky to be in the position of having this support network in place with skills and resources to offer assistance financially, physically, spiritually, and emotionally. So, I leaned in when and where I had the capacity to support. I did this by offering emotional support individually, as well as teaching DBT[1] crisis skills to groups via online platforms.

My hope for the future is that this will be a transformative moment that will radicalize people. It's become clear that we can't go back to the way things were before this pandemic. I hope to see a larger commitment in leftist spaces to focusing on genuine community-building, mutual aid, holistic healing practices, and greater accessibility to members of all communities in their area.

RADICAL MULTI-RECIPROCATIVE CARE: POLITICS OF, POETICS OF, RELATIONS OF INGAT

A poet, community artist and editor at Locked Horn Press who lives as an uninvited migrant settler on unceded Coast

Salish Territories, specifically Qayqayt First Nation (New Westminster), Hari Alluri (he/him/siya) is the author of *The Flayed City* (Kaya Press).

Under Covid-19 restrictions, I've taken most solace (and joy!) in the multi-reciprocation that's happened between my overlapping communities. I'm thinking of: homies checking-in online or briefly at the back-yard alley. Grocery support. Writing groups and events. The Digital Sala, "an intentionally in flux, open-ended, decentralized, messy, but also organized, radically flexible, contingent, & principled experiment of a FILIPINX LIT+ FESTIVAL." Community Building Art Works, The Poetic Record, Letters in Quarantine, BIPOC Writing Community. Ritual and sharing circles. A Rhizome Café-esque birthday party. Loose and woven community I didn't know I was dreaming of before this began. Forms of kapwa I didn't know could happen in this way. Homies and formerly-not-yet-homies becoming part of an impromptu network of support not just to each other but to our communities through each other: nourishment.

And, nurturance: I'm thinking of the homie yelling "Ingaaaat" in our living room just before quarantine and how I now feel that moment as prophecy. At its base, ingat is a way of saying to each other, *take care*, but in the way some of my communities have been using it, it's also a commitment to be part of that care. It carries *remember*. It carries *plan*. It carries *attentive*. It carries *come back*. Ingat is what has saved me and those I love in this crisis. It's what I hope will carry into the post-quarantine world. I believe in ingat. And, through the care, the remembering, the planning, the attentiveness of others, through the coming back – human and non-human, explicit and implicit – it's what believes in *we*.

POEM WITH NO REFERENCE TO MISSING ROOFTOP BACKGAMMON

Social distancing is like a junkyard
superhero, which is to say it does its best
work unseen. That slow picking through

for what might return to the world
at large, that mountain of every name
I will not touch. Which is to say, it's messy out here

even with these emptier streets. As in: among the
 detritus,
a burning disguise. Not the super hero's but of those of
 us
who admit we need that saving. Here is a piece of my

disguise you can burn: I don't need your help.
Here, another disguise – my writing's lie – to feed
the fire: I do it alone. I don't know how far it is

from my junkyard to yours, but I'll approximate
a calculation. Take the hard-won
melody a bass line hungers for, multiply it

by the hunger in a zoo. Not for food – the zookeeper
feeds regular – for the hunting of food. Or the hunt
at all. Even if you're one of those animals

used to being treated as a meal by an animal
in another cage: your hunger for after
the chase, the surprise of your own breath. How, if you
  did

escape the zoo, find yourself in – of all
jungles – a junkyard, you might peek
around the bent parts of a metal mountain,

look across the fire of a burning disguise,
and yearn to singe even a little of your fur
to remind yourself the smell of this place.
              (After Taylor Mali/for the CBAW Crew)

"WE NEED TO FOLLOW THE PEOPLE WHO ARE MOST AFFECTED": NORTH BAY ORGANIZING PROJECT, SONOMA COUNTY, CALIFORNIA
Dani Burlison

As California began seeing its first coronavirus cases and
as shelter-in-place orders came down from the governor,
the North Bay Organizing Project (NBOP) already had
the framework in place to facilitate mutual aid for their
community.

Founded in 2010, NBOP originally set out to address
issues of immigration in Sonoma County. The county
has a large population of immigrants – both documented

and uncdocumented – who do the hard work of keeping things afloat in "Wine Country." Through community engagement and listening campaigns, NBOP's mission then expanded to organize around issues of transit equity and neighborhood development. Over the past decade, NBOP has been praised for its role as a "grassroots, multi-racial, and multi-issue organization comprised of over twenty-two faith, environmental, labor, student, and community-based organizations."

"Cultural strategy is a big part of what we do," says NBOP co-founder and Executive Director Susan Shaw. "We believe culture precedes structural change."

NBOP operates numerous culturally centered mutual aid projects, all of them beneficial to folks during the pandemic. The Rapid Response Network counters Immigration and ICE[2] raids in immigrant communities. The network operates a 24-hour hotline for immigrants facing raids, dispatches legal observers, provides legal defense, and offers accompaniment to victims and families following a raid. The Sanación del Pueblo project started to center undocumented students in response to Trump's threats of rescinding DACA in 2017. Following the fires that devastated the region, the project quickly shifted to also include survivors. The events were offered monthly until the pandemic closed everyone indoors.

"We had everything from herbal consultations, yoga workshops, massage, counselling; we had limpia, a traditional Mexican healing," says Vasquez. "What Susan said about that cultural strategy piece, that culture is at the center of collective care and we were really drawing upon that. That's always been a part of marginalized peoples' culture."

Since the coronavirus crept into the community, NBOP has provided Sanación del Pueblo offerings – herbal classes, yoga and art classes, and instructions on acupressure and more – all online.

"We really need to make sure that mutual aids gets politicized," says Vasquez.

NBOP has multiple taskforces working on centering community leadership and protecting the rights and lifting up residents around the county. One project is Undocufund, a program that Shaw refers to as a community-led redistribution of wealth. The program began as a response to the region's undocumented workers losing wages and homes – and being left out of fedcral emergency funding because of immigration status – during the 2017 fires.

"The money for Undocufund came from over 8,000 people," says Shaw. "It was a lot of little checks and people having events and artists doing events and people selling food; all kinds of creative responses."

Since the pandemic, Undocufund has expanded their focus from supporting fire survivors to also include those impacted by the economy coming to a near halt because of shelter-in-place orders.

NBOP's Housing Taskforce is pushing for the Sonoma County Board of Supervisors to adopt anti-eviction and anti-foreclosure debt relief policy soon.

The Housing Taskforce is also currently working on trainings for the public so renters can learn how to organize ahead of local coronavirus-related "Cancel the Rent" actions.

"You can't, as a random person, just say: I'm gonna cancel my rent. You have to be protected by being together with your neighbors and your community in order for it to be effective."

The trainings are a key component of how NBOP shows up for the community. It is critical in a region that in recent years has experienced simultaneous rent spikes and loss of available housing because of fires. This is a critical moment to bring these changes to fruition.

"The economy that is standing on barely nothing right now is only able to function because of essential workers … they've been undervalued and exploited for so fucking long," says Vasquez. "Capitalism is failing very publicly."

"For the first time, many people are seeing their common interests with everyone else, and seeing this massive failure of the system," adds Shaw. "It's an incredibly painful reminder of what we've done to the earth. But we also see many bright spots of mutual aid and solidarity. There's some sense that we need each other and we're gonna have to figure out how to help each other. We need to follow the people who are most affected, recognizing that they're the ones that need to lead these initiatives."

DIRT, SEEDS, AND SOLIDARITY: TEACHERS ORGANIZING AUTONOMOUSLY FOR FOOD SECURITY
With Nate Freiburger and KT Gunvalson

In late March, an autonomous solidarity project was launched in Northeast Portland, Oregon, to address the food insecurity exacerbated by the outbreak of Covid-

19. La Colectiva de la Comida is a collaboration between teachers, parents, community members, local organizations, the school garden and a local farm. We spoke with two teacher-organizers, Stephen Gunvalson and Stephen White, and Praxis Farm.

Describe your school and neighborhood.
SG: Rigler Elementary is a K-5 Title I school and many people in our community struggle with access to food and basic necessities even when there's not a global pandemic. Our students are multilingual (mainly Spanish and English, as well as several Mayan languages: Yucateco, Akateko, K'iche, Q'anjob'al). Some students are the only English speakers in their household.
SW: Our neighborhood includes several mobile home parks, and where we've focused a lot of attention, especially with online distance learning and trying to connect resources to students who are not only in food deserts but also connectivity deserts. Some folks don't have a phone signal let alone internet signal. That's the context we're organizing in.

How did La Colectiva de la Comida start?
SG: Portland Public Schools announced on March 12th that March 13th would be the last day of school, so we knew we needed to use that day to prepare to support our students during the closure. I immediately created a mutual aid Google survey to gather basic information about the students' families' needs.
SW: We quickly found that food security was a top priority. This project was that visceral response. It's that "oh shit, we have to do something *now*." The work

started how food donations normally work: food banks and overstock from grocery stores and people generously giving from their own pantries. Because of Covid we use lots of caution gathering supplies, and we're redistributing them specifically to the folks at the mobile home parks, which are hundreds and hundreds of people. The work has also been working with other teachers to identify the most extreme need in terms of food insecurity and creating personalized deliveries directly to those families.

What is the future of this project?
SW: We want to move towards more of an agricultural context for the food. We don't know exactly what that will look like and it'll probably be multiple things, especially if our families become leaders and collaborators and farm with us. We hope that farming will be an experience of different worlds in a common space: like the Zapatistas' "un mundo donde quepan muchos mundos" (a world where many worlds fit).

PF: Working with donations from the community and from our CSA [Community Support Agriculture] members, we're building a Solidarity Gardens project, helping folks grow their own food, as well as a quarter-acre Solidarity Field where we're growing crops specifically for free distribution through La Colectiva.

What does solidarity, mutual aid and autonomy mean for La Colectiva?
SW: While we work parallel to the school programs, we're really concerned with creating autonomous spaces where we can have control over our own food and not rely

on food systems that are neoliberal or driven by capital. The institutions have so many other concerns, like preserving themselves and their power, and they're concerned with maintaining the systems and the pathways of power that insulate them from vulnerability and liability. We're working to organize from the margins of all power systems. Our desire is to create something that will last; something that brings people together, that's autonomous, and that no one can take away, that no one can leverage for personal gain. We're walking down a different path, and that path has to do with dirt and seeds and sun and shared meals and solidarity.

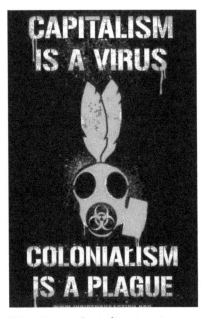

Figure 12.1   Capitalism is a virus, colonialism is a plague. (Photo by Klee Benally)

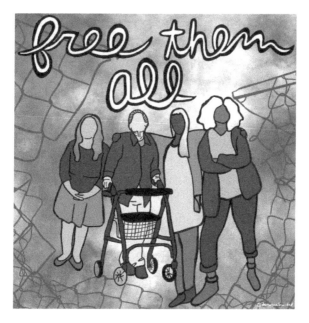

Figure 12.2 Free them all. (Photo by Monica Trinidad)

FREE THEM ALL! PRISONER SOLIDARITY AND ABOLITION IN THE PANDEMIC
Ariella Patchen

Prisoner solidarity and abolitionist organizers on the inside and the outside have been calling attention to the extreme impact of the pandemic on folks who are locked up. We talked with organizers in New York, Michigan and Ohio about the urgent call to free them all.

Maura, NYC, Metropolitan Anarchist Coordinating Council (MACC) and the David Campbell Support Committee (DCSC)

The DCSC formed in January 2018 when David became a political prisoner for protesting the alt-right. The legal work was already well-organized through MACC, so we decided we needed to have our own support committee to organize letter writing, visitations, and the website.

David briefly organized a strike for proper cleaning supplies and we immediately published the demands. People doing this work were like "How can we support?" When coronavirus started it was a chance to continue organizing with No New Jails. We've been applying pressure to the DA offices and local officials by coordinating call-in campaigns advocating for the health and safety of incarcerated individuals on Rikers. We want them to know people on the outside are watching. *All eyes are on.*

Working with organizers is like, *of course you guys are doing this. To sit back and know that all these relationships I have built are reliable and are as serious as I am. That's what virtual solidarity is.*

Now is a time for people to watch the world unravel and see who's there. Like when you go through a personal struggle, you remember the people who were there for you. Anarchist and abolitionist organizers are well-equipped to do work that relies on tools we create ourselves, outside the state. My people and comrades have always been fighting for a better world and always will be. Radical imagination is not being ashamed of these ideas. They're not so utopian that you can only share them in a book or writing.

*Alejo Stark, Michigan, Michigan Abolition and Prisoner
Solidarity (MAPS) and Rustbelt Abolition Radio (RAR)*

MAPS emerged in the wake of the 2016 nationwide
prison strike. Our focus that year was to support those
immediately facing retaliation for striking on the
inside. We slowly started supporting other prisoner
self-activity and organizing on the inside. RAR formed
as an independent but parallel collective to MAPS. As
a movement-building media project, we also support
abolitionist comrades on the inside, interweaving their
analysis, thoughts, and experiences with those outside.

In March we got news from a comrade, Bruce X, at
Macomb, a prison just North of Detroit, saying "Look
the virus is already in here … They have to take immediate measures now."

Two weeks later, Bruce tested positive, and was put
on quarantine. Quarantine means solitary. So here is
this 34-year-old asthmatic – who has been telling us
that this was going to happen – sitting in a solitary cell,
literally gasping for air. We're seeing this tragedy unfold
right before us.

Our immediate response was to put out the interview
along with demands and activate our support network.
Abolitionist comrades with Free Toxic Prisons heard
the interview and immediately organized a phone zap.
The demands were to release everybody over age 50, the
immunocompromised, the pregnant, and those with
health problems as well as free phone calls and com-
missary. But we aren't just relying on the goodwill of

prison authorities. We've also fundraised over $2000 to aid those inside.

A challenge has been to sustain struggle through a sense of grief and impotence. Though it is also the case that what some thought were impossible is suddenly possible. Hundreds are being released in Michigan ... thousands in the US and across the world. As we talked about in a recent RAR episode, using the Zapatista metaphor – there are cracks in their walls – but we still need to pierce through them. We not only have to re-imagine how we should live, but we also have to organize the necessary alliances to collectively pierce through their walls. There's no easy way out, because we are still caught in that building.

Dkéama and Mia, Ohio, Columbus Freedom Coalition and FreeThemAll614

D: The Columbus Freedom Coalition came out of the outrage after Julius Tate Jr. was murdered by Officer Eric Richards.

D: We decided to rebrand the Freedom Coalition and make our abolitionist vision more apparent. We work for freedom for all under a police state, and that means abolishing it.

M: That goes into the FreeThemAll614 campaign, which is about not leaving anyone behind and getting everyone out of jails and prisons.

D: We've been working with law students, Showing Up for Racial Justice, and Mutual Aid Central Ohio.

D: We have four working groups: strategy, aftercare, direct support, and social media. It's probably the quickest I've seen a group come together.

M: We're more connected than we've been before.

D: I think about how we can still prioritize care on a personal level. There's a lot of grief and mourning that needs to be addressed, and a need for rest. The more space for that the more strategic we can be.

D&M: The hardest part is not being in the same room. It's really difficult not sharing space or hugging.

D: It's inspiring to connect struggles in ways that weren't necessarily happening before. There's a lot of optimism, even in this fucked up moment.

M: There's also been people involved who don't want to go back to distant engagement. I've seen different groups saying "Ohio's not going back."

D: I'm trying to build a horizontal world, which starts with building relationships with your neighbors, talking with them … trying to be creative in this moment.

M: I'm excited to see statements like "by any means necessary" not come off as radical anymore. *Just thinking about what is necessary for our freedom, and now it's like no … the word necessary means that it's for everyone.*

D: I remember the first community pride that we had in Columbus. *How it felt there is how I want a horizontal world to be, where we're all free to feel. People just looking after each other, people just happy, gay, and warm.*

FEMINIST SOLIDARITY WITH …

Based in Oaxaca, Mexico, COJUDIDI is the Colectiva Jurídica por la Dignidad Disidente. This autonomous group of compañeras who are psychologists and lawyers provides legal advice and personal support for women facing all kinds of violence, from violence in private spaces to the violence perpetrated by the state and the legal system. In mid-April, magalí rabasa spoke with two members of the legal team: Niza Yek Chávez, from a Zapotec community in Oaxaca, and Mariana Karina Patrón Hernández, from the Valles Centrales of Oaxaca.

How has your work changed since the quarantine began?
N: It changed significantly because our work is all about witnessing and accompanying face-to-face.
M: It's been very difficult to be in contact with our participants who live with their abusers, because they might know what's happening and that can lead to further abuse. We've been developing a safety protocol for our participants, but it's hard to connect because many don't have a computer or wi-fi. But here in Oaxaca we've had the opportunity to weave networks, we have sisters who are psychologists and lawyers who we're in contact with; there's a sense of "I help you" and "I go to your rescue." Those ways of building community have served us in this context.

How did your recent solidarity campaign with women at the Tanivet prison work?
M: I have a close friend who has a loved one in prison, and we talked about how women's prisons are different, because there are also children inside. Also their visitation is a different kind of connection with the outside, and there are many more needs around personal hygiene. We started having conversations and we

thought, why not collect some basic supplies? Knowing that visitors aren't allowed, and that some never even have visitors in a whole year, and now with the quarantine, it's even worse. So it's about thinking of them, and about how their rights are being violated, because the state isn't taking responsibility. With Covid, we always say: "I take care of myself and I take care of others so this doesn't get worse." So we thought about how we could help them in the pandemic. The plan was as much about not bringing the coronavirus into the prison as it was about bringing them supplies. But not only to one or two, but to all 155 women and the 4 children who are also inside.

That's where the campaign started. It was really moving to see that despite all the precarities that we are experiencing, people were very supportive. It makes us think how rad that we are coming back together as humans, that despite all that's happening, there's that sense of humanity, of embracing and accompanying each other. So we started creating those connections, making a chain of support to deliver 155 personal hygiene supply packets. It was very intense, like you almost forget that there's a pandemic and you realize that we can still create community; despite everything that's happening, not only in Oaxaca but across Mexico and around the world, we are still embracing each other, and we are building community again.

When we entered the prison we saw first-hand how the state doesn't care: many of the guards weren't wearing masks or gloves, they weren't taking basic precautions, and they aren't the ones locked up. It was difficult because you think: how is this happening? Inside we saw what the women are going through: the food is precarious, there's no information. They know there's a pandemic, but not really what's happening around the world. Being there allowed us to say: we've brought you these supplies, representing all of the women who are in solidarity with you. It was a chance to share about what's happening on the outside, to offer information that they didn't have yet because no one can visit them.

We were able to see the situation in the prison system, where it is so clear that it is an obsolete, misogynist system, and we got to see how we can work as much as possible to help end the violence of spaces like that.

N&M: The quarantine is a ticking time bomb because you have prisoners of the state, prisoners of disinformation, and prisoners of their own homes. The different forms of violence are tentacles of the system.

What does solidarity mean in this moment?

N: One of COJUDIDI's key values is community. We try to sustain this network not only with the legal and psychological elements, but also among all of us who have found in feminism a kind of rescue from the many internal and external issues that affect our lives.

M: It's hard not to think about multiculturality in Oaxaca and the impact that Covid is having in the [Indigenous] communities. Many have already closed their entrances and exits, and what does that lead to? The cost of food goods increases, there's no access to basic supplies, etc. But this is also how they take control of their *usos y costumbres* (Indigenous customary law) to defend themselves and say, this is happening and we are practicing an independent politics here. So we see all these practices taking root as this pandemic emerges. N: COJUDIDI is an invitation to let ourselves be carried by the networks that have been in formation over the last few years by women, feminists, the assemblies, and other different communities, because these networks can be more effective than the safety measures of some authority or the government. But more than that, we invite everyone to become informed, to become interested, and learn through social media and networks about independent organizations, but also about groups

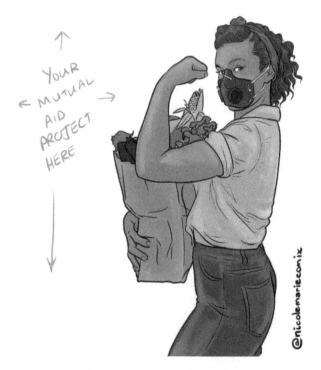

Figure 12.3   Mutual Aid Rosie. (Photo by nicole marie burton)

of feminists, where through the making of community, we help each other.

ARTIST SOLIDARITY: MUTUAL AID ROSIE

nicole marie burton was born in Urbana, IL, to an American mother and Canadian father. She spent her undergrad as a political organizer, student journalist, translator and graphic designer in Vancouver, BC. She currently resides in Ottawa, ON, where she works as a freelance illustrator and a member of the Ad Astra Comix publishing collective.

What made you think to create a poster, the Mutual Aid Rosie?

We founded Ad Astra Comix in 2015, which is a publisher for comics with social justice themes. I am drawn to publishing and movement messaging. So, when Covid-19 hit, a friend who was spearheading a new mutual aid campaign, reached out to me with a simple design idea: something that exemplified the work neighbors were already doing for each other in the wake of the lockdown, but with the spirit of a WWII poster. We settled on a Rosie the Riveter design. But we wanted to keep it relevant, so we chose a woman of color as the hero, and gave her a 3D printed mask. The graphic has been shared over a thousand times online, and I have received photos of the poster being adapted in public spaces around Ottawa, Toronto, Philadelphia, Toledo, London UK, and elsewhere.

What has surprised you most during this time?
I think the speed at which we're all watching, listening, learning, and paying attention to the pandemic as it unfolds. It feels moving to be so psychologically and emotionally present with so many people at the same time – even if we're not all physically "present" with one another. I am noticing that many people who struggled daily with mental health, work, climate anxiety, are doing better than folks who kind of had things "figured out" pre-Covid-19.

Pop culture has been depicting zombies, natural disasters, and social collapse in the media for years, so I've always felt that it – and our enormous appetite for it as consumers – thrived because it was an abstraction of real-world anxieties that were essentially public secrets, but there for us to see if we wanted: climate change and ecosystems collapse, class stratification and the resulting neglect of public institutions and social decay. I grew up squarely within this zeitgeist and therefore feel somewhat "at home" with the idea that things are changing drastically and cannot go back to the way that they were. Indeed, our nostalgia for "the good old days" is a dangerous illusion that is already being wielded by society's most reactionary elements.

Do you think any of the networks created will remain beyond the crisis?
Without a doubt. I have noticed a common thread in reflections from Occupy activists. Many wish to tackle the notion that the movement "failed" because the camps all fell apart or were evicted, or that the movement

did not become a cohesive political party or similar institution. Yet a common narrative theme has surfaced: from all camps came relationships, forming and weaving networks, which in turn inspired new life – both in tangible off-shoot projects and political campaigns, and the more intangible progression of Occupy-inspired intellectual debates and cultural values. These fresh new shoots, both of Occupy but categorically Not-Occupy, are far-reaching and uncountable, which is what we can expect from any and all true mass movements. The movement was alive, and then it died, decomposed, and fed other things. I imagine the Covid-19 mutual aid movement will be similar but bigger.

YOUTH REMOTE LEARNING: MUTUAL AID IN HOMESCHOOLING
Seyma Özdemir

Youth Remote Learning (YRL) is an online homeschooling initiative launched by academics in mid-March to connect families needing educational support and individuals with skills to share. Much to the surprise of the creators, it quickly expanded. Over 30 courses are offered for K-12 students, from Introduction to Japanese to "It's just rocket science." In interviews with founder Shamus Khan (Columbia) and contributors Kate Averett (SUNY-Albany) and Meera Deo (Thomas Jefferson School of Law), we discussed open schools and spaces of imagination through and beyond the crisis.

Personal trajectories, unimagined communities

SK: Being queer-identified is very important because I'm within that broader community thinking about chosen family and my commitments to others. I started realizing that with the stay-at-home orders a lot of people would suddenly have an enormous amount of work, and disproportionately that would fall upon women. I thought to myself, there are also probably a lot of people like me with skills to share that live alone. What are the kind of bridges that we could build between those two groups in a really simple unstructured way?

KA: I research gender and sexuality in childhood and the family, and how beliefs about childhood shape the institutions of the family and education. I have a lot of experience working with kids, but primarily in childcare for younger kids. I first found out about YRL before a lot of schools had actually closed, when Shamus Khan tweeted that it would be great if people who don't have kids could remotely help parents with homeschooling in an emergency capacity.

MD: My research is on legal education, and improving the experiences for vulnerable student populations. With the stay-at-home orders, suddenly my kids were going to be with me, since my husband is a medical doctor and is exempt from the orders. I saw the tweet from Shamus Khan about working to support parents, and I immediately promoted that message. If my contribution is to read stories to little kids, it's something my kids can participate in as well.

Revolutionary moments, uncommodified relations

SK: I never could've imagined what this would be. Suddenly we are doing it, like *making the unimaginable real*. What are the little moments of non-capitalism within a capitalist system and how do those moments make the unimaginable real?

MD: Over 95% of the participants are people I've never met, and probably will never meet. It's an opportunity to connect with people I perhaps wouldn't otherwise connect with. My research has always focused on vulnerable populations. And I think all of us are vulnerable right now.

KA: This experience we are going through together is so rare; this is affecting everybody, so there's this sort of relatability. Every family with school-aged kids is having to figure out what to do. The flip side of knowing that we're living through something we never imagined is that it opens up the idea of what else we could do that we've never imagined!

RELATIONSHIPS AND "DISTANCED" TENANT ORGANIZING

Daniela Aiello is a writer and researcher organizing for housing justice in both Vancouver (on Musqueam, Squamish and Tsleil-waututh lands), as a volunteer with the SRO Collaborative, and in Atlanta, Georgia, with the Housing Justice League for the past six years. The SRO Collaborative was established in 2015 to organize against evictions and for dignified housing in Vancouver's Downtown Eastside and Chinatown. SROs are hotels with small single rooms (typically 10x10) with a shared bathroom per floor, and typically without a shared kitchen.

How has the work of the SRO Collaborative been impacted by Covid-19?
So much of the work SRO-C does is peer-based and tenant-led, in close relationships with constant door-to-door check-ins, collective research, labor, and gatherings – so this time has been challenging. This is especially true for our TOROs (tenant overdose response organizers) and Right to Remain tenants (research group) because they can't come to the office to take active part in the work – such as making kits for safe IV and smoking use. All of that is being done by volunteers and aside from two folks, everyone works from home now. We are working hard to resource as many of the private SROs with harm reduction and hygiene supplies – even buildings we've never organized in. But everything is flipped, which is contrary to our mission. All outreach and relationship building now happens much more quickly and over the phone, but that's only possible because of long-term intimate networks based on trust within and beyond the group. The SRO Collaborative wouldn't have been able to transform the organization and begin this new logistical outreach, including taking on many more buildings, if it wasn't for the last five years of building – networks, knowledge and trust.

The tenants SRO-C works are all ages ranging from late 20s to 65+, majority men, but also lots of amazing women. Many are involved in drug use and trade, most folks are on social assistance or disability. All of them live in a congregate housing setting where people cannot self-isolate or adhere to Covid guidelines in meaningful ways. About 30–45 percent of the tenants in SROs are Indigenous – so those folks are highly over-represented in the neighborhood and more likely to be in precarious housing or unhoused. Many folks move between the SROs and sleeping outside frequently – so it can be a blurry line between housed and unhoused – never mind dignified housing.

There has been a huge spike in overdoses that is a secondary effect of Covid due to the global quarantine efforts, border and trade disruptions among other factors. The drug trade has been seriously disrupted, and many buildings are putting in bad policies, such as no-guests, forcing people to use alone more frequently. It has left a lot of people really vulnerable and the reality is that the drug poisoning crisis is even more of a threat to folks than Covid is at the moment.

During the pandemic you've accepted more donations and funding from corporations, what's that like?
We engage with it because the need is so great, and with all the supply-chain problems (hand sanitizer, spray bottles, etc.) it can be really hard to acquire this stuff right now. We have had many amazing donations, such as 55 gallon barrels of hand sanitizer paid for by fundraisers, LUSH donated 5000 bars of soap. It's a weird version of mutual aid, but it's working and helping people. Though sometimes donations can cause more work to make sure they are suited to the folks we are working with. We had a donation of a bunch of very

fancy smartphones, for instance, and folks need the internet and phones badly right now to stay connected and get help. So we want to accept that, but also giving some folks very valuable items can make them vulnerable to being robbed, etc. So we eventually got some more appropriate phones, and some that work well for folks who are older, and so on. But it was constant tech troubleshooting, and having to make them as low barrier as possible in order for it to all work.

What's been most inspiring?
While there's always been a crisis here, between the drug supply and lack of safe housing, Covid is another devastating layer. The urgency of this hit everyone ferociously, and we have all had to work together more than ever before. So, given that, I have witnessed so much stretching across groups, individuals, and spaces where there have historically been long-standing fissures or differences. There is a lot of incredible collaboration, and people are showing up and fucking working together. So, maybe the mutual aid and solidarity is this coming together across differences – and to me that is something inspiring.

WE ARE ALL PART OF THE SAME CITY, THE SAME HEARTBEAT THAT IS UNIQUELY DC

Eleanor Goldfield is a creative activist, organizer and journalist based in Washington, DC. Growing up partially in Sweden, physical distancing was built in. But she misses hugs so she's giving lots of air hugs to her fellow comrades.

Describe DC Mutual Aid's activities since the beginning of the pandemic.

DC Mutual Aid is a women of color led effort that grew out of existing networks of mutual aid and grassroots organizing to respond to the pandemic. We've set up a hotline to take requests from community members, a place to sanitize and pack goods and then deliver those to our neighbors. DC Mutual Aid is split up by wards and while each ward's workflow is autonomous, we're all part of the same city that is uniquely DC. We're scrappy and underfunded but like all mutual aid efforts, we roll with what comes. As my friend Maurice Cook puts it, "when the systems fail, the people show up." And people really have shown up – proving in spotlit contrast the uselessness of the state. We're constantly changing our protocols, for instance setting up emergency delivery protocols to address dire needs between scheduled delivery days, working to get folks fresh food by building relationships with local, small scale farmers who have been hit hard by the downturn in farmers' market access and restaurant purchases.

How did the collective adapt to this situation?

We've been following the Mutual Aid Disaster Relief Guidelines on safety. It's an ongoing puzzle about how to physically distance when packing supplies. We have sanitation stations set up making it as safe as possible for the folks we deliver to, many of whom are immuno-compromised and/or high risk. But, it is hard to not be able to hug comrades – we're finding ways to support each other while still practicing safe distancing.

Is your work based on any specific principles?
We've based our principles on existing ideas such as the Jemez principles and the democratic confederalism practiced in Rojava. And, we recognize that each place and time is different and no two mutual aid groups are the same. We hold to the ideas of solidarity rather than charity, we never work with police, law enforcement or any other architects of our oppression. We seek to destroy those constructs, using mutual aid not only as a weapon against the designed attacks of capitalism but as a foundation for a new future on the other side of this crisis.

As noted, capitalism is the crisis – coronavirus is just a passing storm. Mutual aid in DC, and elsewhere, has always been there to work with and for those hardest hit by both passing storms and the underlying crisis of capitalism. What's new about this time is that mutual aid is now a global response to the same global storm.

What has been most inspiring? Most challenging?
I knew the system would fail us and let this pandemic creep through our communities unchecked. I knew that the people would show up because that's what we do. What has been really inspiring about that is how creative and powerful these underfunded groups of neighbors have been in getting shit done. As a frontline activist, you see some of the worst sides of humanity – and at the same time, you see the best. It's truly the full spectrum. And I can feel that beauty glimmering – from all over the world. That is my inspiration, my hope. It's always challenging to know that there's more need than we can fully address at any given moment.

Any last thoughts?

The needs will not dissipate, they'll only change. We're hashing out questions with our neighbors: how do we solidify this work of solidarity into real long-term alternatives? There is not one answer – there are millions. And we're excited by these possibilities, always growing, changing, and adapting. We're imagining a continuation of these networks – planning for the adaptation of our work to fight the urge to go back to their "normal" – that toxic normalcy that shanked human rights, that drowned justice and destroyed symbiotic aid. Fuck that normal. To quote a dear friend, Black Panther Kiilu Nyasha: "All Power to the People is not a saying, it's an action. And fighting for liberation liberates oneself."

PUNKS WITH LUNCH: MUTUAL AID AND HARM REDUCTION

Anni is a core volunteer with the mutual aid group West Oakland Punks With Lunch (PWL), which for about five years has been providing food, hygiene, first aid and harm reduction supplies to folks in West Oakland, most of whom live in encampments. In Anni's words, "Cooperation, autonomous communities, compassion, mutual care, inclusivity, a DIY ethos, imperfection, and fun are all at the heart of what we do."

How has the work of PWL been impacted by Covid-19?
When Covid happened we immediately started making big changes about how we interact with our participants, who are a very vulnerable population when it comes to

health. Being unhoused, being stressed and in a state of crisis or trauma, using certain drugs: these all compromise the immune system. And many of our participants are elderly or have underlying health problems. And, of course, living on the street means that you have less control over your space, your access to bathroom facilities, where and how your food is prepared, etc.

One of our first steps was to start bagging all of our supplies into "kits." Before, folks could choose what they wanted: this involved us asking the participants a lot of questions and often getting into conversations. Now, to limit the amount of face-to-face time, we bag everything and participants can choose from the kits: hygiene, wound care, safer sex, safer injection, safer smoking, overdose reversal, menstruation supplies, pet food, and lunches. To maintain social distancing, these kits are dropped in bins at encampments or pushed across a six-foot table to our participants at distribution sites.

We started meeting every day online to figure out protocols to best protect ourselves and our participants. We've put a lot of thought into this and we're still working on improving our practices. We've also tried to share these practices with other mutual aid groups. It's been frustrating to see well-meaning folks walk into encampments without masks or gloves with platters of unpackaged food. I totally understand their desire to help their unhoused neighbors and I want them to continue to find ways to provide mutual aid, but it seems like they don't understand the situation they are putting their neighbors in. Being sick in a house is a lot different than being sick in a tent.

We are collaborating a lot more with other groups who have a history of serving people who are unhoused. In the past, some have been very focused on sober encampments or families and haven't been interested in including people who use drugs in their efforts. But now we see these groups reaching out to us to unite our efforts and ask our help in providing harm reduction to the people they work with.

What has been most challenging?
The biggest challenge has been not being able to really talk with or hug our participants. People who are unhoused or use drugs are already often treated as if they are untouchable and worthless by our culture. A big part of what we try to do is to let folks know that we care about them and that we see them: they matter, they are loved, they are part of our community. Now we have to keep distant, spend as little time as possible with them, spray sanitizer everywhere, and wear gloves. We still try to let them know that we love them and that we are taking these precautions to protect us all, but it's hard. They can't even see us smile because of the masks.

What has been most inspiring?
Seeing how quickly so many people stepped away from the capitalist grind and into mutual aid and community care has been inspiring for me. We've all been faced with a very scary moment, and for so many people, their response has been, "How can I help those around me?" It reminds me that the revolution will happen at home, in our neighborhoods, and with food.

FROM COMMUNITY BRIGADES TO HOSPITALS:
AUTONOMOUS PRACTICE IN HEALTHCARE

Mandeep Dhillon is a Canadian-born ER doctor who has been working and living in the city of Orizaba, Veracruz, Mexico, for the past ten years. She is also a community organizer and member of an autonomous community health collective, founded in 2014 in the region of Tixtla, Guerrero. The Brigada de Salud Comunitaria 43 was named in honor of the 43 students from the nearby teachers' college in Ayotzinapa who were disappeared in September 2014, just as the brigade was beginning its work. Since the outbreak of Covid-19, she has been unable to travel to Guerrero and has been working in the ER in Orizaba.

How has the pandemic changed your work in the hospital? Are you seeing solidarity and mutual aid at play in that institutional context?

Because my organizing efforts had not been put into that hospital environment until now, it's been a bit of a strange experience, but also interesting in terms of creating closer bonds between doctors and nurses and orderlies where there's usually quite a split imposed around class lines. Right now folks working in the hospitals are feeling quite vulnerable. Interestingly, it's been one of the only experiences where as doctors, you have to think about how treating someone may affect your own health. That particular new feeling associated with our work is sort of opening us up to understanding that other sectors that work in the hospital are also vulnerable, and so that's been something positive.

On my shift we've been doing skill-sharing with the nurses and orderlies, getting ready for patients with Covid, because the hospital isn't providing us with any of that information. A lot of strategies we're learning come from folks in New York and other places that have already been hit, and we're trying hard to share that kind of knowledge with other workers in the hospital. That's been one of the parts I hope will set a precedent for later. Of course, in these crisis moments it can go either way and it can force people to just become more selfish around their own rights, but I'm hoping that at least in some cases it will open up more communication between all these different sectors that are working in the hospitals.

All of a sudden we've had really beautiful points of solidarity in terms of getting 3D-printed gear from one of the local universities. A few weeks ago, when it was looking really bad in terms of the equipment that we were going to have I started reaching out to friends and one of the professors at the Instituto Tecnológico de Orizaba got in touch with me and we started working on 3D-printing face shields for the hospital, and then word got out and they got asked by a bunch of other clinics and hospitals and it's been really awesome. He said that it's been really nice because forever they've worked as an insular unit and haven't had this ability to connect with "real issues," as he put it, outside of the university. It's really opened up relationships that usually don't exist.

How do you think this experience can shape approaches to health in the future?

One of the things I've been feeling quite intensely, and I think it's because of my background as an organizer, is this incredible sense of urgency that I feel to get back to community health organizing. The experience of Covid has made really clear to me what the Brigada's work opened up for me, which is that autonomous health structures and health-related organizing is the way we need to move forward. We know that the fact that health institutions have been completely gutted by neoliberal policies has facilitated the way that this pandemic has happened and who it's affecting in particular. But I think we can take another step to prioritize other ways of thinking about health. A couple months ago we were in Tixtla in a workshop and I was telling the compas that we need to visualize scenarios where folks won't even be able to move from their communities, and how do we get ready for that? At the time I was thinking about repression. I wasn't even thinking about a pandemic and I never thought that this kind of situation would come so quickly. It's made it really evident how necessary it is to have folks trained and prepared for all sorts of scenarios. And for that reliance on the government and official institutions to be lowered for us to be able to take care of ourselves in more meaningful ways.

NOTES

1. Dialectical Behavioral Therapy (DBT) is a form of psycho-therapy rooted in holistic wellness, and I have been using my access to free DBT training (via a scholarship) to redistribute these skills to others in my communities.
2. Immigration and Customs Enforcement.

PART VI

South America (Argentina and Brazil)

CHAPTER THIRTEEN

Argentina: Injustices Magnified; Memories of Resistance Reactivated

Nancy Viviana Piñeiro and Liz Mason-Deese

March 24th is a day of commemoration, struggle and mourning in Argentina. The mourning of our +30,000 disappeared during the last military-civilian-economic dictatorship, which began on that day in 1976, is usually expressed through marching. Hundreds of thousands of people take to the streets across the country. This year, on March 24, people were forced to remain in their homes – those who have one – while the gendarmes were on the streets. For all the Argentinians and Indigenous peoples of Argentina for whom social justice and memory is an important part of their lives, not being able to take to the streets – for this or any other cause – is experienced as a kind of collective impotence.

But creativity and willpower always overcome: thousands of people across the country put up signs on their windows, doors and balconies that read "NUNCA MÁS" (Never Again) or "30,000 detained-disappeared present!"

A strict shelter-in-place order was enacted in Argentina on March 20, meaning residents are only allowed out for a

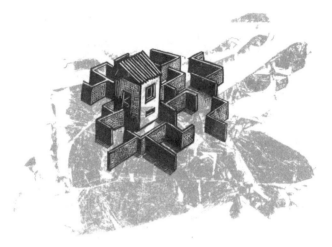

Figure 13.1 Hogar artwork. Monocopy print with nylon and xylography. (Artist: María del Mar Mayo. @Tallerdeexperiment acionvisual)

small set of exceptions, such as purchasing food or medication or working in vital services. While the government attempts to implement emergency social and economic measures, it is hampered by the country's looming foreign debt and its obligations to international creditors, and the public health system has been devastated by years of neoliberal policies at the request of those same creditors. Meanwhile, coming after two years of economic recession, for many people staying home means not being able to buy food or pay the rent, especially for the 50 percent of the country that works in the informal economy.

The police and the gendarmes enforce the quarantine through violence, especially against black and brown, and poor bodies, but of course not everyone has a safe home to stay in. In the slums of Buenos Aires and other major cities, extended families often share living spaces, including kitchens and bathrooms, making social distancing difficult. To give one example among many, Villa 31, a slum in the center of Buenos Aires, directly in front of one of the city's most expensive and luxurious hotels, went weeks without running water, making basic hygiene impossible, and quickening the spread of the virus through the neighborhood. Women and LGBTQI people face particular risks as confinement leads to increased domestic and care duties, and greater chances of violence. So far during the quarantine, there has been an average of one femicide per day in the country.

However, much about this crisis is not new for Argentina. Grassroots social movements, neighborhood assemblies, and all kinds of networks have long developed ways of responding to economic and social crises. In the midst of the economic crisis at the beginning of the millennium, people established robust solidarity economies, including barter networks and alternative currencies, and worker-managed cooperatives, while movements self-organized soup kitchens, schools and health clinics. These economies were essential in enabling people to survive the crisis and even sustain the subsequent "economic recovery" largely based on widespread precarious labor. Even before the pandemic hit, many thousands of people around the country regularly relied on these self-organized soup kitchens for their meals, and on all kinds of mutual aid networks.

We believe it is necessary to keep reactivating our memory of resistance, acknowledging the ongoing colonialism and the genocide upon which the nation-state was founded, and that can be seen today in the financial colonialism exercised through the foreign debt, while strengthening our own networks. Extraordinary times like these prove that the tools we have built for ourselves and the lessons we have learned are our reservoirs. This memory of solidarity from below under the pandemic seeks to be a contribution to those tools.

* * *

By Nancy Viviana Piñeiro

CARE FOR THE ROOTS: EARLY CHILDHOOD AND FAMILY SUPPORT DURING THE PANDEMIC

I know M. She and her partner welcomed me in their home in the province of Mendoza back in 2016. M is a teacher, a psychomotor skills and early childhood development specialist, and the principal of a preschool for children from two months to three years old, located in one of the many poor neighborhoods sprawled across our country. Beautiful as they are, I can't give M's real name nor even the kindergarten's, because they are disobeying the Ministry's orders with regards to the educational materials sent as "homework," a constant source of stress for families and educators. One does not readily associate disobedience with teachers. Knowledge, love, care? Yes. But could disobedience and even rebellion be a necessary element in teaching, could it actually nurture?

I remember M in her chaotic backyard full of plants. She's slender, with dark long hair, gentle but vivacious in her gestures. It is as if I could almost see her when I read her reflections. She writes to me in an outburst.

I feel pretty good, although sometimes I'm devastated, angry. Inequality comes to light even more so now, I mean, in a simultaneous, multiple way, augmented, like a huge magnifying glass. We work in a marginalized urban neighborhood, gradually transformed through the countless crises from a place of rural and factory workers, to mostly unemployed families who do off jobs. In the worst areas, families in makeshift houses made of wooden sticks, adobe, mud or black plastic bags, try to make ends meet without drinking water, sewage or gas supply. "Stay at home" is a very difficult command for them.

I ask M how she copes with those feelings, what her "tools" are.

Being a witness to this affects me, these are not mere facts, it makes me feel there is little one can do in this extraordinary circumstance where struggling alongside others is more limited. But I recover my strength partly because I have been part of several networks for more than twenty years. And I work at a kindergarden that we founded 27 years ago with a group of teachers and neighbors. We are six teachers and six teaching assistants.

Such networks have made this a very special place.

The space is very precarious in terms of the resources provided by the state and the working conditions. Administratively, the school is "private," but there's no tuition fee. We managed to build a lot of autonomy. Even if we keep demanding the state give us what they should, we are committed to our project, we sustain a community-based pedagogical proposal guided by a respect for children and their families. We hold weekly assembly meetings with the teachers where everyone's word circulates: their feelings, their views, among a diversity of ways of life and even ideologies.

I come to learn of the preschool's situation through M's Facebook posts. After the suspension of classes, there is a first priority – how to keep feeding the children and helping the families. The municipal government sent them food packages.

Beginning on March 16th, we collectively decided to organize a "food watch," taking turns to go to the school to distribute the packages. We had to make our own masks. The government sent us the list of the 70 people who should receive the food packages, but there were only 25 packages with the bare minimum. We had to tell the families: "You are not on the list." I made two videos on that day and shared them on social media. A community radio called us, we made this visible, but so far there is no solution from the state.

M and the teachers decided to find ways to bring food for all the families. They ended up feeding them with much more than that: tenderness, listening, even music.

So many people offered their help, some of them are artists (and they don't have money to spare! On the contrary). We asked them if they could send us songs for the families, the other fundamental aspect of sustenance, which is art. It became a spontaneous virtual network where some are sending us lullabies, beautiful, tender, caring. Each teacher selects and decides what to send and to whom, it's not just about sending stuff. It's about feeding with art, fostering tenderness.

So what about the other food?

We received donations from neighbors, socio-environmental assemblies, and also vegetables (half were donated, and half bought) from agroecological producers. You know, in this terrible situation where many people don't have access to food, small producers are being paid pennies, they either bury their squashes or throw them to the pigs. We had some money from donations and thought, why not reach out to them? We paid them twice what they were getting. That's part of the way we want to think. Thinking to be able to act.

I ask M how they felt in this rushed but conscious task of organizing.

I think we feel potent or impotent depending on how well we can respond to the situations. We want to do more than what the bureaucracy mandates; it's a shared feeling of satisfaction. One day the teachers told me they had decided to disobey the Ministry of Education's criteria for the learning materials during quarantine: they weren't relevant. It was more important to open spaces of dialogue, not harass them with activities. Thus we began getting more feedback, more engagement. The curriculum is a relationship. A quality relationship between the children and the adults.

We keep learning how to be educators even during a pandemic, establishing relationships of solidarity and reciprocity where there is an implicit way of being and doing with the other. Our ongoing shared struggles are our "reservoir." But I don't know exactly how to preserve ourselves, to resist the destruction of so many lives and create alternatives. I have many questions.

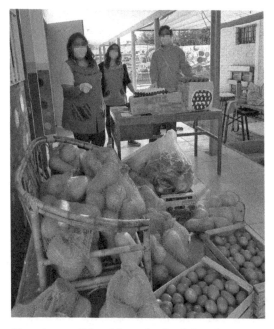

Figure 13.2   School, base for food distribution.

BEGINNING AGAIN WITH QUESTIONS

As I reflect on this collective project and its many geographies and histories, I think about the impossibility of emancipating our imaginations without acknowledging and redressing the genocides of the past. As a country built upon the genocide of the Indigenous peoples, I decide to reach out to Lefxaru, a friend from the Lof (community) Newen Mapu, in the Argentine Patagonia. I want him to be part of this. He sends a few lines and thoughts. He's brief and wise as usual. But what I didn't know then was that his words would echo M's:

There are people who share their certainties with us, but also, and this is key, they share their questions, their doubts …

Our experience is sustained essentially through the questions we ask ourselves …

Those questions that mobilize, break maps, open paths …

Those people who build strength in uncertainty – with them I go to life and I go to war, I go to death and to the party, with them I plunge into a river or a song …

THE "OTHER FUNDAMENTAL ASPECT OF SUSTENANCE"

I did not say this at the beginning, but during this pandemic I am stuck in New York, I cannot return home yet, flights have been cancelled. María del Mar shares on social media a watercolor painting using natural pigments of wine, turmeric, everyday elements. I am desperate to do watercolor and have no paints yet. I write to her and thank her for that inspiration. María is an arts teacher in the city of Buenos Aires, she articulates with other artists in her workshop, which I came across through another artist. They form a loose network based on principles of collaboration as opposed to competition. And she is also a member of Submundo, a collective of artists who are currently at risk of losing their place since they cannot pay rent. I think about M again and her words. María del Mar comes to mind. This is how their color, from seemingly different palettes, complement each other:

> I want to talk about cultural productions – maybe shifting the focus away from the word "art." We need to realize that this is a tool for structuring our thought processes, opening channels of communication. I'm arguing with those who say that art is useless or that the only important thing is having a roof over our heads and food. It is fundamental, but what gives meaning to our lives is not only that. Art also makes visible our contemporary political problems, whether it's dance, literature, painting.
>
> As a school teacher I see that institutionally we're not reflecting on what's happening right now. As for arts classes, they haven't modified the contents, they asked us to proceed as "normal." In this situation of confinement, I think our need to explore our own world becomes evident. Drawing, painting, music, listening, literature bring us to this other rhythm, to a different mode of observations. That is the tool. It helps us

observe, conceptualize, express. We can find in this a meaning or not: exploration for its own sake, without any utilitarian result. Sit down, observe a plant, draw it. See how the leaf pattern resembles our veins?

Cultural creations should have the place they deserve in our mental health, in becoming a person, in building empathy.

May we be worthy of the task. May we take the plunge together.

*   *   *

By Liz Mason-Deese

AMPLIFYING VOICES

We are the type of people who are left out of emergency plans. Foreign bodies. We are the waste of a society that treats us as second class citizens under any circumstances, discarded. For them, we are the virus.

Thus opens a statement from the collective YoNoFui in the early days of the pandemic in Argentina. YoNoFui is a feminist and popular political organization made up of women and non-binary people, some of whom have been previously incarcerated. The organization was founded in 2002 and organizes art, communications and skills workshops inside and outside prisons and also operates a worker-managed textile cooperative, publishes a regular magazine and hosts a weekly radio show.

The collective's political practice is fundamentally situated in the back and forth between inside and outside of the prison walls. With each of our actions and proposals, we seek to question the prison as an institution, to place value on those life trajectories as another type of knowledge among other unique knowledges, within a horizon of social transformation. The composition of YoNoFui is heterogeneous and interdisciplinary in terms of know-hows and life trajectories. The collective is made up of sewing workers, militants, activists, housewives, market vendors, students, visual artists, dance and theater artists, poets, teachers, and designers.

All of these different knowledges and know-hows, skills and capacities have been put to work when responding to the coronavirus crisis. I ask them how the pandemic has affected incarcerated people in Argentina.

The pandemic rendered visible the terrible conditions of confinement for those who have been deprived of their freedom in our prisons, especially the women and children. There are no state policies to care for that population. On the other hand, the pandemic brought the overcrowding and overpopulation to a true social explosion. With the appearance of Covid-19, requests for house arrest increased and, at the same time, life within the prisons became increasingly unbearable after the quarantine was decreed and visitation prohibited. The detained people started going hungry, and with the hunger, revolts began demanding sanitary measures, food, and hygiene products that are generally provided by visiting family members. On the other hand, prison staff did not respect the protocols, they would come and go without taking any care to avoid exposing the entire prison population to the risk of contagion. Today the debate has polarized, there are rumors of strikes in the prisons, it is an ongoing conflict.

As conditions inside prisons become increasingly unbearable, YoNoFui has worked with other organizations to conduct surveys of which prisoners have the greatest health risks and which are eligible for early parole. They emphasize that many of those women were arrested for minor drug trafficking offenses, essentially a form of criminalizing poverty. Meanwhile, right-wing groups launch a media offensive claiming that the government is going to release murderers and rapists and thousands of people take to their balconies banging pots and pans *against* the release of prisoners.

The way in which the hegemonic media spreads misinformation about house arrests and possibilities of parole causes impotence. This issue is being treated in a completely hostile, cruel, and stigmatizing way, once again we are characterized as the internal enemy, the terrorist. This causes us distress but it also activates our potential to struggle. In the face of so much explicit fascism, we are forced to seek strategies to construct collectively, to challenge how the media produces hateful subjectivities. We have to change those narratives and amplify our voices to make known what are the true circumstances that we are experiencing.

ACCOMPANIMENT NOT CHARITY

YoNoFui has built on its existing networks in order to organize mutual aid for women under house arrest and formerly incarcerated women, many of whom work in the informal economy and now have no way to earn an income because of the quarantine.

During the health emergency, we have faced several emergency situations, one of them was accompanying the compañeres who are going through a very difficult material and economic moment, especially those who are under house arrest. Many compañeres live in small rooms with their children who cannot go out to play, this situation is very difficult and distressing, others are self-employed and facing dire economic circumstances. The worst situations are of those women who have to spend quarantine with a violent partner. In the collective, we are doing everything possible to accompany each one of those different experiences.

Based on those situations, we have been carrying out collections and requesting donations through social media and our different communication channels. With the proceeds we buy food and hygiene products that we distribute to the compañeres who are in very serious situations aggravated by the context of the pandemic. We have had to create specific strategies to reach the different points of the city of Buenos Aires and the metropolitan region, dealing with the restrictions on transit during the obligatory social isolation. So far, we have presented more than 100 families with bags of food and cleaning supplies.

We were already engaged in mutual aid prior to the pandemic. Currently, some features are intensified, but accompanying each like this has always been part of our everyday political practice.

LISTENING BECOMES A FUNDAMENTAL SPACE

Despite the fact that it is difficult for many compañeres to keep up constant virtual communication, due to lack of resources or unfavorable conditions of time and space, we maintain contact with them. We carry out collective activities and exercises through WhatsApp groups, sharing perceptions and feelings about what we are going through. It is not easy, but given the conditions of isolation, it is the only way that we have to be close to and accompany one another. Our job is to accompany these realities and together compose spaces and experiences that allow us to transform our lives collectively.

It causes a lot of anxiety to receive messages from the compañeres who are inside, they call us every day and it is difficult to transmit calm or any certainty about their issues and desires. At the same time, listening becomes a fundamental space. The ambiguity of co-existing emotions offers us a scenario that is both catastrophic and, on the other hand, invites us to rethink everything, to think about other ways of creating a non-patriarchal justice. We already know that confinement is not a solution, that prisons only function as places to store bodies. Now that this problem is becoming more clear, it is also a moment for opening up the imaginary and raising demands that seemed unthinkable, such as the abolition of the prison system or a universal basic income, an income that would allow us to take a break from capital. Therefore, we carry out specific actions to survive day to day and we also give ourselves spaces for debate and discussion to find a breathable future.

We understand that mutual aid can take different forms, and while it is important to obtain food, clothing, hygiene products, it is also important to strengthen our practices of listening. The situation within the prison walls is increasingly unlivable, there are no longer any activities, visitation has been cancelled, and there is great uncertainty. In this context, being able to talk about feelings, about fears and anxieties, having the feeling that someone is listening from a place of love, brings a lot of calm. Reinforcing these networks is fundamental, networks that are alternatives to the state, that are rooted in feminisms and movements of dissident sexualities. Questions arise such as: What does self-care mean? What are we caring for and how? It is important that it not be the state that monopolizes care because that renders invisible years of work that organizations have been doing. We understand that no one saves themselves alone, this idea that staying at home alone is a way of saving others seems very problematic to us. There are many of us who are taking risks to continue reinforcing these networks, because we don't believe in "armchair individualism," because we know that the solutions are always collective.

CHAPTER FOURTEEN

On Grassroots Organizing: Excerpts from Brazil

Vanessa Zettler

We agreed not to die. (Conceição Evaristo)

When the pandemic hit, Brazil was in the throes of an ultra-conservative movement, reified in Jair Bolsonaro's presidency. It's been a political scenario representing a backlash against human rights so jarring that its rhetoric includes open endorsements of old policies from the military dictatorship era of Brazil (1964–85).

Minorities have been under even more violent attack. At the same time, labor rights are under threat, there's been a record percentage rise in precarious jobs. In 2019, the percentage of informal workers among the employed population was 41 percent, according to the Brazilian Institute of Geography and Statistics. And it was in the midst of this drastic political scenario that, by the end of February, there was the first confirmation of Covid-19.

In a country marked by extreme social differences, with the second highest concentration of wealth on the planet, the tragedy of class divide started shaping the story of the pandemic right away.

One of the first deaths, the third one registered, was of a poor, 63-year-old woman who worked as a maid for a family in one of the wealthiest neighborhoods in the city of Rio de Janeiro. Her bosses had arrived from a trip to Europe infected with the virus, but had her continue to work in their house. They recovered, she didn't.

Entire neighborhoods had no water coming out of their sinks, while the media was telling them to wash their hands. People living in cramped houses were told to socially isolate themselves. #Stayhome hashtags flew around, while thousands of homeless people wandered the streets. The public health system, SUS, was now endorsed and cheered everywhere as our possible savior, but only after years of regressive policies and reformations that took investment away from it.

On April 29, Brazil registered 5,017 confirmed deaths, surpassing the number of losses in China. "So what? What do you want me to do? I don't work miracles" was the answer of President Bolsonaro when asked by a journalist about these numbers. To make matters worse, these numbers are underreported, for there is a tremendous shortage of tests.

The year of 2013 will always be remembered for the massive demonstrations for social advancements that took place in the country. We saw the rise of the conservative movement coming right after it and channelling into this genocidal government. Nonetheless, people have never stopped grassroots organizing.

Here, I interview people who have had ongoing engagement with different forms of local organizing. People of color, people in the peripheries of the big cities, Indigenous people, people of the land, women. People for whom Covid-19 is not the first threat to their ways and means of life. People who have resisted and built communities for centuries in order to survive and thrive. It is a snapshot of a specific area of Brazil, the non-centric areas in the densest cities in the country, São Paulo and Rio de Janeiro. It's also a snapshot of how these people's work has proved to be so essential for the creation of realities that generate hope.

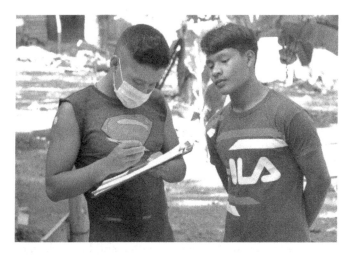

Figure 14.1   Indigenous community in Jaragua. (Photo by Richard Wera Poty)

A local bar in the neighborhood of Campo Limpo, on the peripheries of São Paulo, once turned into a weekly open mic in 2004, brought together local poets, musicians and cultural agitators. Suzi de Aguiar Soares, 53, and her husband, Binho, don't have the bar anymore, but "Sarau do Binho" (Binho's Open Mic) has become a reference point for peripheral literature and arts. It has now also become a hub to fight Covid-19, being central in organizing a large network of solidarity.

As soon as the corona started, there was great distress. So we started putting material on the web. Our poetry and music, with the hashtag #SarauemTemposdeCorona (Open mic in the times of Corona), ignited people to also send videos, which grew a lot. That became therapeutic, providing many people space to feel better. I think that through art we can heal some wounds, help people who are sad. Poetry is a form of healing.

We also started a fundraiser along with other local collectives in the area. We have already been able to help more than a thousand families in the region, way before government aid arrived. We have been part of a very large network, and that just makes it grow bigger.

The way I started it was by calling people and checking how they were. Solidarity is about asking: How are you? How can I help?

There are people who do not express their need for help. There are people who are just depressed ... A friend of mine, for example, a writer, with 4 children, told me she couldn't get out of bed. She had recently stopped teaching at school to live off her writing. And so she has no prospect of work and she was lying in bed. I talked to her, sent her money, and then she went to buy food, sent me a photo and told me "Suzi, this is so much that I can still share with two more families." And she did. There was a woman who received the 300 reais we sent to her, she took R$25.00 out of that and donated it back to our fund, because she wanted to help too. It is beautiful to see how these acts of solidarity activate people, make people stand up and do something for someone too. It is very important to take care of people's self-esteem, and that is how solidarity spreads.

Now we are seeing which side people are on. New connections are emerging between groups and people, which we are organizing through WhatsApp, and we are now the Covid Combat Support Network.

In Rio de Janeiro, André de Carvalho, 48, has lived his entire life in favela Morro da Formiga. Son of migrant workers, he became an organizer in 2013, a watershed moment in his life, having seen the possibility of working for social transformation with his own hands.

Morro is a place of resistance, a quilombo. I am proud to be from here, for it made me who I am. There is an invisible wall that separates the asphalt from the favela. The work I do here happens through creating connections between these worlds.

We, residents of the favelas, know what our demands are. When the pandemic started the concern of the people here was whether they would be able to eat or not.

At that moment, though, we had a lot of partnerships, people sent money here, donations of food and basic supplies ... Another gap has been the issue of education. We are, therefore, focusing on making people understand the seriousness of the moment. This is a very hard job because our people have a lot on their heads, and it's been hard for many to understand you can't socialize like before anymore.

There is a deficit in education in the territory of the favelas, and we know it is a project which allows people to be manipulated by discourses such as the one of this president. So we spread audio messages, stencil, graffiti, music, rap, funk. Every kind of tool possible to send a message speaking to the very reality of people.

Solidarity for me is a basic principle for us to live in a harmonious way. It is the opposite of social chaos.

I am hopeful that if there is anything good that we can get out of this pandemic, it is to weave new networks of people acting together for the common good.

Conjunto da Maré is a large area of many favelas in Rio de Janeiro, with 140,000 inhabitants. Timo Bartholl, originally from Germany, moved there in 2008, living in and part of grassroots collectives ever since. He is part of collective "Roça!" which produces agroecology and operates as a community space. From the beginning of the pandemic he has been organizing with the recently formed Frente de mobilização da Maré.

In the favela, whenever there is an emergency, it leads to an expansion of networks.

The Maré Mobilization Front is one of those. We operate on three axes: economic support, communication, and self-care. There are no tests for those who are not hospitalized by SUS. Right now we are making an online form to try to find out which families suspect cases so that we can at least make some projection.

We have a very big problem of disbelief in the media, so communicators are using social networks to speak to residents, adapting the information to the reality of the favela. For example, here there are people who don't have water at home. So we put up banners saying "If you have water in your house, share it with those who don't."

I see that people are keeping an eye on each other. People warn us, they say, "Look, my neighbor has no job, I think she needs food supply," that kind of thing.

A lot of people here work in the informal sector. Many, for example, make a living selling snacks and drinks in traffic jams. So, from one day to the next there is no more source of income, because there is no more traffic jam. At this moment, support between social classes has become even more important, and people have sent money here.

As time goes by, I want to see what international solidarity will look like.

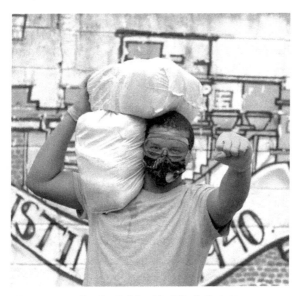

Figure 14.2   Favela da Maré in Rio de Janeiro.
(Photo by Davi Marcos – frente de mobilizacao mare)

Helena Silvestre has been an activist for her entire life. She lives in the south of the city of São Paulo. There, among many other projects, she started the Abya Yala Feminist School. A place where women organize locally and build what Helena calls a "favelada feminism."

The Abya Yala Feminist School is a permanent challenge: to build, from favela women, a feminism that expresses and embraces what we are, with our trajectory of black diasporas, indigenous genocides, expulsion from the land and reconstruction of community in violated territories such as favelas and peripheries.

As we are rooted in territories that never existed free from hunger, our first thought when the pandemic hit was: women will not be able to stay at home while their families are in need. We immediately started an organizing process between us, shared tasks, mapped women in extreme situations, mapped volunteer women with a car and mapped food donors. From those first deliveries, the mental health alert rang: many grateful women received food baskets and told us, sometimes crying, the story of how they were on the edge. So we started to organize psychological assistance at a distance with two psychologists who are part of the Abya Yala, building protocols and procedures. The psychological assistance reinforced another debate, which is the situation of domestic violence with women locked up with their aggressors. Hence, this was another front established with some ideas that we are trying to produce as minimal support networks for women who are in suffering like this.

Our adaptation has been difficult. But what inspires me is to hear from women who are totally vulnerable that they want to help in some way. As the number of assisted women is growing a lot, several say they didn't know groups such as ours existed, and say that they want to be part of it, sewing masks with donated fabrics that we take, and helping as they can.

I think that with this pandemic, we realize that privileges are always a dynamic relationship and if we, as favela inhabitants, have no privilege in relation to women of the white and college educated middle classes, in having a home and guaranteed work we are in a privileged situation in relation to other sisters who need our attention.

Solidarity is an action and not a discourse, it's a rooted and everyday construction. This makes it possible to eliminate the myopia that only sees politics in the "extraordinary acts of the hero." It also allows those who want to change the world to change themselves first.

In the north of the city of São Paulo there is a Guarani Indigenous land, Aldeia Jaraguá. Thiago Karai Djekupe's family has been fighting for the right to stay on the land for generations and to protect the native nature that surrounds it.

We were occupying a land near our territory to defend it from real estate investments as the pandemic hit, and so we went back to our community and started working on prevention right away.

The first thing we needed to do was to isolate ourselves from the outside world. Since we are in São Paulo, isolation was very hard since here we depend on white people's economy to survive.

So corona arrived to our territory. Today we have two confirmed cases, and other suspected ones.

We are demanding fast testing for everyone in the community. So far we've had a few losses of indigenous people to corona in other territories throughout Brazil. We are part of the Guarani Yvyrupa Comission that covers the Guarani people from all territories, and the APIB, which is the Articulation of the Indigenous People of Brazil. Through these organizations we exchange information and organize to work for prevention and to denounce abuses.

We've been saying this for a long time. That if human kind continues treating mother Earth the way it has, mother Earth would try to get rid of it. We knew it was coming.

I find it hard to believe that Juruás (white people) will really understand that it is necessary to change their habits. That it is necessary to respect and get to know the elderly, that we need to be wise, to live in solidarity, to respect the youth ... I think Juruás forget very fast.

In the capitalist model of civilization it is hard to learn to live in equilibrium.

Even after suffering so much, once things get better, people forget. People have been under so much anxiety that their way of life has imposed on them that they take risks, because without risking their lives they can't survive in that system.

People are still confused about who they are. Ailton Krenak, my godfather, indigenous leader and author, wrote about this lesson we learn from the elderly: postponing the end of the world will take people re-learning how to live. Understanding that simplicity is what matters. That having shelter, food, joy and community is what one needs, so we can have an actual sustainable life. This life is possible, but Capital has been fighting this idea and this model of life since its beginning. Capitalism is trying to destroy our indigenous culture as another way to destroy this model of a communal and sustainable life.

A movement that has been subverting the colonial distribution of land in Brazil for the past 35 years, and one of the largest social movements in Latin America, the Landless Movement, the Movimento dos Trabalhadors sem Terra (MST) operates through the occupations of vast areas of land, putting it into agricultural production, while demanding land reform. During the pandemic, they have been very busy distributing this production to people in need. Maria Alves is a farmer and educator in the MST, active throughout her 66 years. She told me how this movement has brought her and many others their dignity in being field workers and to work for the abundance of life on the planet.

From the first time I saw a march of the MST I knew where I wanted to be. We value mother earth and everything it provides. I work in the production sector here at Comuna da Terra Irmã Alberta, an occupation just 30 km away from the city of São Paulo.

Brazilian people eat very badly. It is a shame that our country applies so much pesticides in food production. We insist on the importance of a healthy and diverse diet in three daily meals. But now with the pandemic, we know many people won't have it. This is a shame. A country of fertile land, with so many natural resources, is not supposed to have anyone hungry.

The MST is making donations to those who need it. We do what we can. People contribute some money. These amounts become purchases from MST farmers, and the produce is distributed. It brought tears to my eyes to see how much the families were in need, and how much we were able to help. This is happening all over Brazil, in the various areas where we have food production, we are distributing in a very organized way. We are not alone. We see many other networks and movements doing this. That is very uplifting.

I think this is one more event, another moment that helps us to reflect deeply on everything. The democratization of land must be in the countryside and in the city, so that everyone has access to the wealth of this country. We must be together with indigenous movements, quilombolas, urban movements. We are all defending life.

People will start to reflect a lot about solidarity. They will start to consider: "who's on our side? Who do we have to defend? Who are our enemies?"

I think that in the end it can have an awakening effect on people.

To strengthen the people, so they recognize themselves and take pride in who they are.

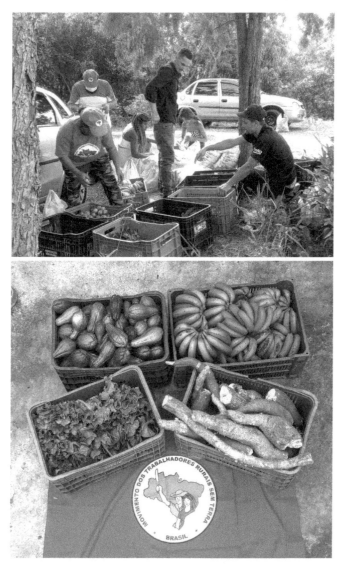

Figures 14.3 and 14.4 From the MST food distribution.
(Photos by Raul Miranda)

We have to do a job that it seemed like we were not able to do until people saw this evil all over the world. I feel very much like this ... wanting this pandemic to end as soon as possible so we can resume all the work we have to do again.

And it has to be collective, participatory and cooperative.

Concluding to Begin

Dear Reader,

This is a story without an end.

For many, this Covid-19 pandemic is just the most recent disaster in a longer history of crisis, struggle and self-organization. We acknowledge and express our gratitude for those who came before us and to all those who continue with these transformative projects.

If you are reading this, you yourself have likely done something to care for others, perhaps simply by wearing a mask or shopping for a neighbor. In our many different ways, we are already participating in a tapestry of care and mutual aid that spans across the globe.

So, we end this book with an invitation to reflect on, amplify and join together in this work.

Above all, we close these pages with love.

In solidarity/solidaridad/bi piştgirî/solidarietá/同舟共濟/
solidariedade/Dayanışmayla/ एकजुटता में/dlúthpháirtíocht
ngokubumbana/σε αλληλεγγύη /بالتضامن/ پشتگیری /
연대의 마음을 담아

Colectiva Sembrar

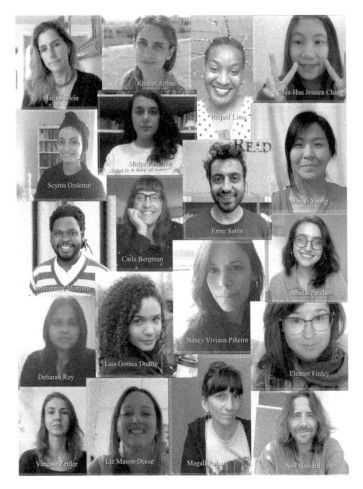

Author photo collage by Ferit Ozdemir

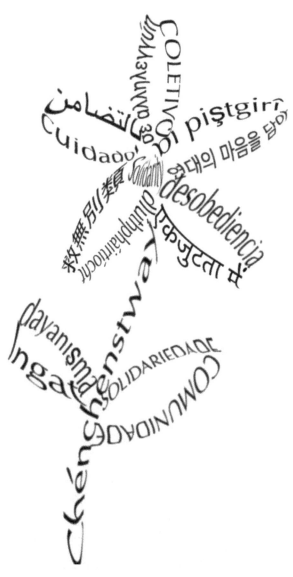

Flower image/drawing by Ariella Patchen

Notes on Contributors

Khabat Abbas is an independent journalist and video producer based in Rojava. She has extensively covered developments in Syria; from the creation of women's organizations to running alongside frontline fighters in battles against ISIS and witnessing the devastating moments of the more recent Turkish occupation. She has published in local media outlets and produced for influential foreign media. Khabat also has experience in the humanitarian field serving at MSF and currently UNHCR in projects aiming to assist internally displaced persons and refugees. Her personal interests include women's empowerment, culture and mythology, as well as Kurdish music and folklore.

carla bergman is a mom, an independent scholar, filmmaker, and budding poet. She is the co-author of *Joyful Militancy*, and edited *Radiant Voices: 21 Feminist Essays for Rising Up*. The threads that run through all her work are: radical social change, and amplifying voices and acts of solidarity and autonomy at the edges. carla spends much of her time capturing beauty with a camera, and walking with her partner, kids, and friends on Tsleil-Waututh, Squamish, and Musqueam Lands (Vancouver, BC).

Chia-Hsu Jessica Chang is a doctoral candidate in Comparative Literature at Binghamton University. Her recent interests are the politics of de-naming and re-naming, the technologized body and Asia as method.

Lais Duarte is a Ph.D candidate at the Anthropology department of CUNY. She studies solidarity networks, immigrant integration policy and decolonisation praxis. Lais is also a proud pet mama and spends her days dreaming of and fighting for a socially equitable and loving world.

Eleanor Finley is an activist-anthropologist at the University of Massachusetts, Amherst, an editor at *ROAR Magazine*, and a former board member for the Institute for Social Ecology. She has been writing political ethnography since Occupy Wall Street and conducted activist-research about climate activism, social ecology and the Kurdish freedom movement. Her dissertation explores the practice of direct democracy within the European Kurdish diaspora. She lives in Friuli Venezia-Giulia, Italy.

Neil Howard is an academic (and) activist based at the University of Bath, in the UK. His research looks at exploitation, marginalization and how/whether unconditional basic income and non-violent community organizing can help overcome both. He is engaged with a variety of social movements, co-parents two children, and desperately longs for a world where the meeting of needs takes priority over the making of money.

Han Gil Jang is a writer, visual artist and translator currently based in Seoul. His current interests range from Asian diaspora art and the East Asian postwar experimental avant-garde to memory and representation of war.

Midya Khuduhur is a Fulbright Scholar with a master's degree in Comparative Literature from the State University of New York-Binghamton. Since 2014 she has been involved with humanitarian organizations and UN agencies and has four years' experience dealing with Syrian refugees and Iraqi displaced people who were affected by the ISIS attacks. In 2018 she returned to academia to do her master's, and subsequently gained a keen interest in Kurdish Studies especially Kurdish literature and cinema.

Raquel Lima is a poet, art-educator and Ph.D candidate in Post-colonialisms and Global Citizenship from the Centre for Social Studies at Coimbra University, where she works on orature, slavery and afrodiasporic movements. She is also an anti-racist activist and loves crossroads.

Liz Mason-Deese is a translator, researcher, cartographer and feminist activist living in Buenos Aires. She is a member of the *Viewpoint Magazine* editorial collective and the Counter-Cartographies Collective.

Boaventura Monjane is a Mozambican postdoctoral researcher at the Institute for Poverty, Land and Agrarian Studies (PLAAS, UWC) and fellow at the International Research Group on Authoritarianism and Counter-strategies of the Rosa Luxemburg Foundation.

Nancy Piñeiro Moreno is an Argentine militant translator and interpreter, grateful that her engagement in counter-hegemonic translation for social and political change is continuously keeping her from finishing her Latin American Studies MA thesis.

Seyma Özdemir is a Ph.D student at SUNY Binghamton. Her research interests are international migration, political economy, cultural studies and feminist theories. Nowadays, she is talking about capitalism with her children, drawing pictures, making laboratories, trailers, puzzles out of cardboard, imagining better futures and creating new spaces with them in quarantine.

EP & TP are involved in anti-authoritarian assemblies in Greece.

Ariella Patchen is a student, artist, activist and dreamer located in Binghamton, New York. She aspires to write about and participate in social movements across the world, as she imagines what it means to build a revolutionary new world.

magalí rabasa lives in Portland, Oregon with her partner and two kids. She is the author of *The Book in Movement: Autonomous Politics and the Lettered City Underground*, as well as numerous articles about independent media networks and autonomous movements. Over the past two decades she has participated in various alternative media, popular education, and radical publishing projects across the Americas. She is currently an assistant professor of Latin American cultural studies at Lewis & Clark College, where she encourages and incites critical conversations and actions related to the settler-colonial identity of the institution.

Debarati Roy is a Ph.D student at SUNY Binghamton's English program where she focuses on South Asian cinema and literature, minority narratives and diaspora studies. She is a Humanities New York Public Humanities Fellow (2019–20). Her project, titled "Untold Stories and Diasporic Voices," documents the migrant experiences of the South Asian diasporic community in the New York area. Through film screenings, exhibits and roundtable sessions, her project engages with untold stories of migration, belonging, and social and cultural mobility.

Emre Sahin is a participant and researcher of social movements, particularly the Kurdish movement, and a sociologist at Binghamton University. Until the Covid-19 pandemic, he was writing his dissertation on prefigurative mobilization and revolutionary transformation in Rojava. Recently, he has been nurturing non-human forms of life and thinking about the impact of consensus-seeking in decision-making processes.

Marina Sitrin writes about, and participant in, societies in movement. She is a professor at Binghamton University, a mother and dreams of a free world. She is the author of *Horizontalism: Voices of Popular Power in Argentina*; *Everyday Revolutions: Horizontalism and Autonomy in Argentina*; the co-author of *They Can't Represent US!: Reinventing Democracy from Greece to Occupy*; and the forthcoming *The New Revolutions from Social Movements to Societies in Movement*.

Ji Young Shin is an assistant professor at the College of Liberal Arts, Yonsei University. Her current research involves examining the changes in East Asian minority communes circa 1945 from the textual studies perspective. Ji Young is also a member of RefugeeXField and Wednesday Peace Studies Group, where she strives for the liberation of refugees, women, people with disabilities and animals altogether.

Rebecca Solnit is the author of more than twenty books on feminism, western and indigenous history, popular power, social change and insurrection, wandering and walking, hope and disaster, including *Whose Story Is This?*, *Call Them By Their True Names*, *Cinderella Liberator*, *Men Explain Things to Me*, *The Mother of All Questions*, *Hope in the Dark* and her memoir, *Recollections of My Non-existence,* published in 2020.

Vanessa Zettler is a teacher, sociologist, translator and writer. She graduated in Liberal Arts from the New School for Public Engagement, with specialization in Sociology by FESP-SP. During the time she lived in New York, she was part of the group who started the Occupy Movement. Vanessa is Brazilian, currently living in São Paulo where she is also an activist building community through music.

Index

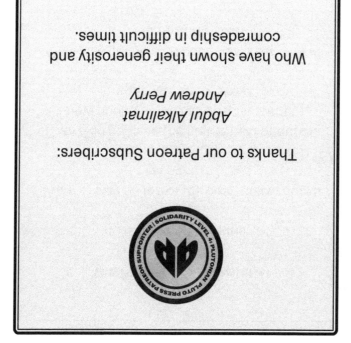

Thanks to our Patreon Subscribers:

Abdul Alkalimat
Andrew Perry

Who have shown their generosity and
comradeship in difficult times.

Check out the other perks you get by subscribing
to our Patreon – visit patreon.com/plutopress.
Subscriptions start from £3 a month.

The Pluto Press Newsletter

Hello friend of Pluto!

Want to stay on top of the best radical books we publish?

Then sign up to be the first to hear about our new books, as well as special events, podcasts and videos.

You'll also get 50% off your first order with us when you sign up.

Come and join us!

Go to bit.ly/PlutoNewsletter